HOW TO MONITOR YOURSELF

Step 1
Know that your doctor needs your expertise
as much as you need hers.

Step 2
Know that you—and only you—can say where it hurts,
how much, and when.

Step 3
Know that without your input, your doctor will have a
much tougher time figuring out why it hurts.

Step 4
Take into your own hands the history of your
health—and a power to protect your well-being that is
nothing short of revolutionary.

In this book, learn about:
- Routine tests and how to read them
- The best health Web sites
- Hospital do's and don'ts
- Doctors' symbols and abbreviations on your chart
- The eighteen symptoms that should send
you straight to the doctor
...and much more.

WHEN IT COMES TO YOUR HEALTH, YOU ARE YOUR OWN KEEPER. FIND OUT NOW...
HOW TO SAVE YOUR OWN LIFE

HOW TO SAVE YOUR OWN LIFE

The Savard System for Managing—and Controlling— Your Health Care

Marie Savard, M.D.
with Sondra Forsyth

WARNER BOOKS

A Time Warner Company

Names and other details in case histories have been changed to protect privacy.

Warner Books, Inc., 1271 Avenue of the Americas, New York, NY 10020
Visit our Web site at www.twbookmark.com

W A Time Warner Company

Printed in the United States of America
First Printing: May 2000
10 9 8 7 6 5 4 3 2 1

Library of Congress Cataloging-in-Publication Data
Savard, Marie, M.D.
    How to save your own life : the Savard system for managing—
and controlling—your health care/ Marie Savard with Sondra Forsyth.
      p. cm.
    ISBN 0-446-67619-5
    1. Medicine, Popular. 2. Self-care, Health. 3. Consumer education.
I. Forsyth, Sondra. II. Title.

RC82 .S268 2000
610—dc21   99-088906

Book design and text composition by Ellen Gleeson
Cover design by Jon Valk
Cover photograph by Blanche Mackey

For my husband, Bradley Fenton, M.D.,
and for our sons,
Zachary, Aaron, and Benjamin

MS, M.D.

For my son and daughter,
Christopher and Stacey

SF

Contents

Acknowledgments   ix

Introduction: Whose Health
Is This, Anyway?   xi

Step 1   Trusting Yourself as the Real Expert
About Your Health   1

Step 2   Collecting and Studying Copies
of Your Medical Records   24

Step 3   Researching Your Conditions,
Diseases, and Injuries   44

Step 4   Learning Which Immunizations,
Exams, and Tests You Need and When   67

Step 5   Helping Your Doctor Help You   115

Step 6   Participating in Decisions About Your
Treatment Options   136

Step 7   Knowing How to Get the Best Care
in the Hospital   153

Step 8   Finding the Courage to Treat
Yourself Right   179

Epilogue: Here's to Your Health!   196

Appendix: Copies of Actual
Medical Records   199

Index   233

About the Author   239

Acknowledgments

I would like to thank my husband, Bradley Fenton, M.D., for his unfailing love and support not only during the writing of this book but always. Zachary, Aaron, and Benjamin, my three sons, deserve my gratitude for their genuine interest in my work—they are simply the best.

A special thanks to Eileen, my sister and business partner, who has given up other professional opportunities to work with me. My six other brothers and sisters read over my early writing as we all huddled together for days outside the intensive care unit, waiting for word about my father. Their comments were invaluable. I also appreciate the help I got from my mother, a retired nurse, and my father who together spent hours reviewing the medical Web sites. *I thank God for giving doctors the wisdom and tools to return my husband and father to good health.*

My best friend Gladys and her husband Dick offered encouragement throughout the research and writing process. Two other dear friends, Marilyn and Tom, helped me believe in the importance of my message—and put up with the fact I monopolized their fax machine every time I came to visit.

Without my literary agent, Loretta Barrett, this book would never have come into being. She heard me speak at our alma mater, the University of Pennsylvania, and encouraged me to pursue my dream. Loretta teamed me with journalist Sondra Forsyth, who immediately "got it." Not only that, but when Sondra played it back to me, the message had become clearer and more powerful than ever. My thanks to her for our wonderful friendship.

My appreciation also goes to my editors, Jamie Raab and Jessica Papin, for their insight and enthusiasm. Finally, my heartfelt thanks to all of my patients over the years. They are the inspiration for everything you are about to read.

Introduction

Whose Health Is This, Anyway?

"If I am not for myself, who will be for me?...
If not now, when?"
—Hillel

You have the power to avoid the pitfalls of modern medicine and get the best possible care. The secret is to do for yourself what your doctor can't do. This means taking charge of your own health. If you're like a lot of my patients, you're surprised by what I'm saying. As one woman put it, "But I thought I was paying *you* to be in charge."

I can sympathize with her. The notion that all you have to do is find a good doctor who will take care of you is definitely comforting. However, my own experience as well as recent research shows that the more you get involved in preventing and managing illness instead of relying on your doctor as a cure-all, the healthier you'll be. But that's not all. These days, the task of coordinating the various aspects of your health care falls to you, not your doctor.

Before you start wishing we could turn back the clock, think about the exciting development that set the changes in motion: Research has yielded breakthrough after breakthrough in diagnostic techniques and treatment options which can help you live longer and feel better. However, the corollary is that while Marcus Welby, M.D. knew just about all there was to know back in his time, your doctor today has no way of being up on every single one of the near-miracle advances that are made almost every day. That's why we have so many specialists now. That is also a compelling reason for becoming an active participant in your own health care.

So much for the upside of the situation. The downside is that the advent of managed care has meant that doctors typically have a "panel" of 1,000 patients or more. In contrast, Marcus Welby had a private practice with a few hundred patients he took care of from cradle to grave. He knew their names, he made house calls, and he kept all their records tucked in his desk drawer. Without even referring to those records, he pretty much remembered who was allergic to penicillin, who was on insulin, who had high blood pressure, who was prone to ear infections, and even who was overdue for a checkup. Today's doctors couldn't possibly keep all of that in mind. Once, when I was in a group practice, I was so swamped and rushed that I found myself wishing I had a snapshot of each patient stapled to the chart to help me recall which person I was about to see! Add to this the fact that people move around a lot these days—kids go away to college, employees get transferred, retirees head for the Sunbelt—and you can see that if anybody is going to keep track of your health history, it's going to be you.

My eight steps will help you do exactly that. The steps work equally well whether you belong to an HMO, whether you have insurance that lets you go "out of network," whether you are one of the 43 million Americans who have no insurance at all, or whether you live in a country which has socialized medicine. Key among those steps is collecting copies of your original medical records and making them available to everyone involved in your care. This may not be the first time you've heard that piece of advice. I mentioned it back in 1996, in *Woman's Day* magazine, and I've seen brief references to the idea in several books since. Yet to my continuing frustration, this indispensable step toward taking control of your health care has never caught on. A dramatic example of that sad fact occurred during the last days of the insolvent HIP Health Plan of New Jersey. As the doors were closing, workers had to deal with scores of panicky patients trying to get ahold of their own records for the first time.

I believe the reason people such as those HIP patients wait until a crisis to get their records is twofold. First, no complete guidelines have been presented until now about precisely how to accomplish this seemingly overwhelming task. And second, the topic has most often been presented as a call to arms *against* the prevailing health care system instead of as a way to work *with* the system. That kind of adversarial advice is not conducive to a collaborative doctor-patient relationship, and people shy away from it. Time and again when I lecture and conduct seminars, I hear people voice a fear of antagonizing doctors and hospital personnel by requesting records. Ironically, however, when I speak to doctors on this topic, they react with unanimous enthusiasm and relief. They understand immediately that patients who collect and study their own records, and who make it their business to become well informed about their health concerns, will be in a position to join forces with doctors instead of either worshipping them or seeing them as the enemy.

What you're about to read in the pages that follow is based on my thirty years of experience first as a nurse, then as an internist both in solo and group practice, and as a legal expert in malpractice cases. During those three decades, the health care system has become increasingly complex and fragmented. The long-standing paradigm of the all-knowing physician as the authority figure in a white coat simply doesn't work anymore. My hope is that this book will usher in a new era in which patients routinely archive their own medical records, have confidence in their instincts, exercise their rights, shoulder the responsibility for prevention and compliance, and enter freely into a fruitful partnership with their doctors. Only then will we move beyond the current health care crisis and go on to achieve optimum well-being as a nation.

Marie Savard, M.D.
June 1999

HOW TO
SAVE YOUR
OWN LIFE

Step 1 Trusting Yourself as the Real Expert About Your Health

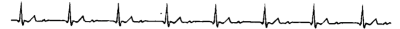

*"Each patient carries his own doctor inside him.
They come to us not knowing that truth. We are at our
best when we give the doctor who resides within
each patient a chance to go to work."*
—Albert Schweitzer, M.D.

The itching began in the middle of a humid summer night. Carol Watkins bolted upright in bed, flicked on the light, and checked for mosquito bites. She had spent the evening on the deck of her condo, sipping a margarita and talking nonstop with her dearest friend about their new status as divorced single moms. The citronella candle hadn't done much good, but the two women ignored the bugs. They were determined to enjoy the lilac-scented breeze and the starry sky. Carol figured she was paying the price. To her surprise, though, there were only a few bites and they weren't where the itching was. It was intense and generalized, making her want to dig at her skin with her nails.

An ominous shiver went through her. Although this was by far the worst episode, Carol had been feeling mildly itchy for several months. She hadn't thought much about it, even when it gradually got worse. Now, though, the words "Something is really wrong with me" popped into her head. She got up and found the calamine lotion. It helped a little and she finally fell into a fitful sleep.

The next morning, the itching was still there. After putting her two daughters on the bus for day camp and driving to her job as an executive secretary at an accounting firm, Carol called her doctor. He told Carol to try a moisturizer, since it sounded as though she had dry skin. Carol hung up the phone and stared out the window for a moment. This time, she said the words out loud: "Something is really wrong with me." The itching had gotten worse and now it was everywhere, a deep and urgent feeling unlike anything she had ever experienced before. Still, the doctor hadn't seemed at all concerned. Carol didn't want to come off like a wimp or a hypochondriac and she reasoned that anybody who had been to medical school must know what he was talking about. Anyway, Carol thought maybe the itching was just psychosomatic. She was having a rough time adjusting to the divorce, especially when she had to drop the kids off at her ex's house and see him with the Other Woman.

A week later, though, Carol gave in and called her doctor again. She felt silly, but she told him the moisturizer hadn't helped. He referred her to a dermatologist. Carol heaved a huge sigh, sure she was going to get some relief at last. The dermatologist couldn't find anything specific, however. But he did prescribe an ointment he thought would take care of the problem.

It didn't. By this time, Carol was going out of her mind trying to take care of the girls and pay attention at work on very little sleep. She tried two more dermatologists and one cream after another, but nothing worked. Eventually, fate stepped in. Carol's employer switched insurance plans. She had to choose a new primary care provider and go for a complete physical. She ran her finger down the list of doctors and picked me.

I first saw Carol Watkins for what I thought would be a routine visit on a burnished September afternoon over a

2

year after her first severe bout with the itching. She was obviously embarrassed to tell me her symptoms. I remember her words well. "It's just itching, but it seems like it comes from inside. I've had kind of a bad year, so maybe this is nerves. But I can't help wondering whether there's something really wrong with me." I put my hands on the lymph nodes on either side of her neck. Experienced fingers can feel even a slight enlargement. Carol's right node was swollen, but it wasn't causing her any pain. I ordered blood tests and then a biopsy of the swollen lymph node, but I was pretty sure I already had my diagnosis: Hodgkin's disease, a type of lymphoma that has a distinctive cancer cell. Pruritus, the medical term for itching, is a common symptom. And at thirty-two, Carol fell into the riskiest age group, fifteen to thirty-four.

The tests and biopsy confirmed my educated guess. Carol turned out to have Stage 1 Hodgkin's, limited to a single node on one side of the body. As I always do with my patients, I gave her copies of the test results and helped her understand them. Her complete blood count (CBC) and blood chemistries were all normal, including her liver tests. This reassured me that she probably didn't have advanced disease. However, her sedimentation rate, at 64, was abnormally elevated. The average for women is about 20. The "sed" rate is a tipoff that something systemic and significant is going on—either inflammation, infection, or cancer. In addition, Carol's biopsy showed the typical cell of Hodgkin's, the Reed-Sternberg cell.

"You're lucky, insofar as anyone with cancer can be called lucky," I said gently. "The prognosis is very good. I'm going to send you to a cancer specialist, an oncologist. In most cases like yours, radiation is all that's needed and the cure rate is high." Carol managed a smile, and put the copies of her results in her purse. "Well, at least now I know what's wrong," she said. "Even though it's not the world's greatest news, I feel better already." Throughout her treatment, she saved all her reports, summaries, and test results and shared all the findings with her radiation specialist and oncologist. She didn't have to repeat her story or worry that they didn't have the information they needed. She was truly at the center of her care, not at the periphery.

There's a happy ending. Radiation cured her, as is true in 90 percent of cases similar to hers. But the lesson here is that Carol could have kept ignoring her own instincts, allowing the cancer to spread and her chances of recovery to lessen. When the itching didn't subside after a few months, she should have made an appointment for a physical with her doctor. Checking the lymph glands is a routine part of any examination and he would surely have made the diagnosis. But like most physicians today, he probably had what we call a "panel" of at least a thousand patients and maybe as many as 2,500 or more. He no doubt left it up to the patients to make and keep their appointments and to communicate with him. I'm not making excuses for him, and it's your judgment call as to whether he should have decided that a year was too long for him to keep giving Carol phone referrals to dermatologists without having a look at her. But the point is that he didn't ask to see her. That left the ball in Carol's court. Yet she was afraid to seem pushy or paranoid and she thought her problem might be all in her head, so she never clearly stated the fact that she suspected something serious was going on.

She's certainly not alone. Most people don't trust their "doctor within." They're too humble for their own good. Yet study after study has shown that patients know much more than they think they do about their own health. For example, researchers at Purdue University tracked seven thousand patients ages twenty-five to seventy-four for twenty years beginning in 1971. Dr. Kenneth Ferraro, a sociology professor, headed a team which had the subjects rate their own health from poor to excellent and fill out a questionnaire about their diseases. Then doctors looked at the patients' self-assessments, did extensive examinations, and wrote their own evaluations. The result? In every case, the patient's own report was as accurate or even more accurate than the physician's was. Or as renowned British physician Sir William Osler put it, "Listen to the patient. He is telling you the diagnosis."

Even so, patients are typically cowed by doctors and other health care professionals. They're afraid to have faith in their own instincts. If that includes you, you're actually making your doctor's job harder. Time and again, I've asked patients what they think might be wrong and they have said, "You tell me. You're the doctor." But studies show that 80 percent of what doctors go on when they make a diagnosis is what patients tell them about their symptoms, history, and lifestyle. Technology is wonderful and we have many sophisticated diagnostic techniques that weren't available even a few years ago. Still, there is no substitute for what *you* know about how *you* feel—and how it is different from the way you usually feel. Believe it.

LISTEN TO YOUR BODY

First, however, you need to give yourself permission to home in on how you feel and get the message. Aches and pains, bleeding you can't explain, the sense that nothing tastes good anymore, tossing and turning all night—whatever doesn't seem quite right to you probably isn't. Your body is smart enough to send you warning signals. All you have to do is pay attention. And if a symptom turns out not to be serious, so much the better. There's nothing embarrassing about telling your doctor you've been seeing blood on the toilet paper, and finding out the cause is hemorrhoids instead of colon cancer. Your doctor will be as pleased as you are with that diagnosis. And it goes without saying that if you do have cancer, you'll be glad you caught the illness early enough that a cure may be possible. In other words, rectal bleeding is not normal. Your body is telling you that something is wrong. Don't dismiss the symptom just because it might be nothing serious.

I am thinking of the very sad case of Steve White. He had what he called "bowel problems" starting in his early thirties. On his honeymoon, he confessed as much to his bride, Cindy. Back home, he went to a doctor and said he was often constipated and occasionally saw some blood. The doctor put him on a high-fiber diet. Cindy did what she could to keep him on it. But by his own admission, Steve cheated a lot. He was a rising stockbroker and he liked his power breakfasts and power lunches, heavy on the eggs and bacon and meat and potatoes. The bowel problems continued, but Steve never went back to the doctor. Why bother, when he knew the trouble was that he wasn't eating the way he should? But on some level, Steve also knew it was more than that. How could a change in his bowel pattern happen when he hadn't changed any of his lifestyle habits? It just didn't seem right.

It wasn't. Fast-forward to a damp April morning five years later. Cindy got a call at the school where she taught third grade and their twins, Amy and Marla, were in kindergarten. Steve had been taken to the emergency room with a dangerously high fever. The doctors on duty were mystified and by the time Cindy got there, Steve had already been admitted. In the days that followed, tests revealed that Steve had colon cancer. The symptom that got him to the hospital has been dubbed "tumor fever." But long before that, Steve had harbored the fear that he wasn't well. Yet he failed to act on that fear. Doctors estimated that Steve's cancer, a slow-growing form, had taken over five years to get to the advanced stage they diagnosed that April. If he had believed his visceral feelings and pressed until he got a diagnostic test called a colonoscopy, polyps could have been detected and excised easily before they became malignant. As it was, Steve's chances didn't look good. And in fact, he died a little over a year later at the age of thirty-eight. True, the doctor Steve originally saw could have ordered a sigmoidoscopy or a colonoscopy, but Steve hadn't sounded all that urgent about his symptoms. Also, there was no family history of colon cancer, and Steve never went back to give his doctor a second chance. The only person who really knew, day in and day out, that something was very much amiss was Steve himself. His body was talking and he wasn't listening.

Here's another story, but one with a positive outcome. Tim O'Connor, age thirty-two, did listen when his body talked. Tim is an avid golfer. One Saturday as he lofted the little white ball a respectable distance into the air, he felt a tearing pain in his groin. His foursome had been walking, but the one behind them had an electric cart. They drove Tim back to the clubhouse. By that time, he was also feeling nauseated. He called his "telenurse," a person assigned by his HMO to field phone calls from patients. She was soothing, but didn't seem to grasp the intensity of the pain or the severity of the problem. She suggested an ice pack. "A guy would have understood," Tim said later, sounding exactly like women who complain that male doctors don't get it about menstrual cramps or labor. In any case, Tim believed his body, not the nurse. He asked his buddies to get him to the ER.

Diagnosis: torsion, or twisting of the right testicle around its own spermatic cord. Because Tim got immediate attention instead of sitting in the clubhouse with an ice pack, his testicle was saved via surgery. Had he waited more than twenty-four hours, with the blood supply to the testicle effectively cut off, he would have lost the testicle. "Sometimes you just have to go with what you know," Tim says.

Amen. Here's a list of eighteen symptoms that should send you straight to the doctor, plus a capsule look at what the best- and worst-case scenarios might be. Remember, there are often plenty of other possibilities, and other symptoms—such as Tim's painful testicle—can be emergencies as well. Frequently, a thorough workup by health care personnel is needed in order to get a diagnosis. But what I want to emphasize is the fact that these eighteen symptoms should not be ignored, since they do sometimes signal serious problems requiring immediate medical attention. I developed this list when I taught a course for acupuncture students about how to recognize the red flags that signal the need for evaluation and possible treatment by a physician trained in Western medicine. I used the standard checklist doctors follow when taking medical histories: the review of systems (ROS). The ROS starts with what are called "constitutional symptoms" such as weight loss and fatigue. Then the ROS literally takes it from the top, working from the head down to the feet:

1) Loss of appetite and weight loss
Best-case scenario: Dieting, elderly with decreased interest in meal preparation, mild depression.

Worst-case scenario: Cancer, liver disease such as hepatitis, severe and possibly suicidal depression, chronic infections such as TB, anorexia nervosa, Crohn's disease.

2) Severe headaches

Best-case scenario: Acute viral infection, tension, migraine.

Worst-case scenario: Sudden onset of your worst headache ever could signal an aneurysm in the brain (thinning of an artery, which may then balloon and rupture). Sudden onset with fever and stiff neck could signal meningitis. Gradual onset with escalating intensity on awakening could signal a brain tumor. The antibiotic minocycline, which is used to treat acne, can cause increased intracranial pressure and blindness if left untreated. This complication is extremely rare.

3) Redness in the white of the eye

Best-case scenario: Conjunctivitis (pink eye) from contagious virus or staph bacteria, or an allergic reaction to pollen or contact lens solution. The eye could also simply be bloodshot from fatigue or alcohol use.

Worst-case scenario: Acute glaucoma or uveitis or a foreign body in the eye. Note that in these instances there will usually also be pain and decreased vision.

4) Persistent cough

Best-case scenario: Postnasal drip, asthma, acid reflux (heartburn), or the vicious cycle of a continued cough caused by irritation from coughing.

Worst-case scenario: Severe asthma, tumor such as lung cancer, lymphoma, heart failure or fluid in the chest. Note: A chest X-ray can help rule out serious problems.

5) Shortness of breath

Best-case scenario: Obesity, sedentary lifestyle, hyperventilation from anxiety.

Worst-case scenario: Sudden onset can signal a pulmonary embolism (blood clot in the lung). If the episode happens while you're lying down or exercising, the cause may be angina (blockage in the arteries, which may result in heart failure). If you have a history of allergies or asthma, this may be a serious asthma attack.

6) Chest pains

Best-case scenario: Esophageal spasm from acid reflux (heartburn), unexplained "stitch," inflammation of lining of lung or rib cartilage.

Worst-case scenario: If the pain is of recent onset and is coming in episodes of five to fifteen minutes each with tightness that doesn't get worse when you breathe deeply but does get worse with exercise, the cause may be angina (see number 5). If you're also experiencing shortness of breath, this could signal a pulmonary embolism (blood clot in the lungs). Other possibilities are a collapsed lung, a dissecting aorta, or an aortic aneurysm.

7) Persistent abdominal cramps or pain

Best-case scenario: Spastic colon, viral infection, intolerance to lactose (a substance found in milk and milk products), gas from beans or from sugar substitutes.

Worst-case scenario: Especially if accompanied by nausea, vomiting, weight loss, and change in bowel habits, the cause could be a tumor, a ruptured organ or ovarian cyst, diverticulitis (inflammation of a diverticulum, or pouch, in the lining of the colon), a gallbladder or pancreas attack.

8) Rectal bleeding

Best-case scenario: Bright red blood on toilet paper or in the bowl is important but can wait until a routine doctor's visit. The cause may be hemorrhoids or a fissure (tear in rectal tissue from straining).

Worst-case scenario: If the blood is black or maroon and tarlike, this is a medical emergency such as a bleeding ulcer, bleeding diverticulitis, or other colon problem, or colon cancer. Note: The iron in vitamin supplements and in certain vegetables can color the stool black. So can Pepto-Bismol.

9) Vaginal bleeding after menopause

Best-case scenario: Atrophic (dry) vagina, irritation from intercourse, side effect of hormone replacement therapy (HRT).

Worst-case scenario: Cancer of the uterus.

10) Pain, lump, thickening, or any change in breast tissue

Best-case scenario: Breast cyst, normal changes during menstrual cycle, infection, or inflammation.

Worst-case scenario: Breast cancer.

11) Frequent episodes of dizziness

Best-case scenario: Inner ear viral infection, naturally low blood pressure (which is good even though it causes the dizziness), or anemia.

Worst-case scenario: Warning of a stroke because of blockage of blood to the brain, heart arrhythmia, heart failure (if accompanied by low blood pressure), or, rarely, acoustic neuroma (a benign tumor which can cause hearing loss unless it is surgically removed).

12) Sudden weakness or numbness of one side of your body

Best-case scenario: Hyperventilation from anxiety, migraine.

Worst-case scenario: If separate episodes lasting less than twenty-four hours occur, this could be the warning sign of impending stroke. If weakness or numbness is persistent, a stroke may have already occurred.

13) Confusion or change in mental or thinking status

Best-case scenario: Mild depression, aging, stress, low blood sugar, or fasting.

Worst-case scenario: Severe depression, brain tumor, adverse drug reaction, drug interaction, or drug overdose.

14) Numbness or pain in feet and legs when walking on inclines

Best-case scenario: Arthritis of spine (stenosis), improper shoes.

Worst-case scenario: Circulatory blockage (claudication), neuropathy from diabetes, or exposure to toxins such as metals, paint, or lead.

15) Jaundice

Best-case scenario: Eating too many carrots or taking too many supplements with carotene.

Worst-case scenario: If accompanied by abdominal pain, this could signal gallstones or a gallbladder infection. Without pain, this could mean a tumor or a viral inflammation of the liver (hepatitis).

16) Changing mole or dark spot on the skin

Best-case scenario: Aging spots called seborrheic or senile keratosis.

Worst-case scenario: Melanoma or other skin cancer.

17) Profuse sweating

Best-case scenario: Anxiety, exertion, hot room, hot flashes, or high fever breaking.

Worst-case scenario: Especially when unexplained and accompanied by a feeling of doom, this could signal a pulmonary embolism (blood clot), a heart attack, or a ruptured aneurysm (see number 2).

18) Insomnia

Best-case scenario: Stress, worrying, uncomfortable mattress, light or noises, caffeine, or side effect of medication.

Worst-case scenario: Severe depression, adverse reaction to medication.

DENIAL IS NOT JUST A RIVER IN EGYPT

Now that I've given you some common warning signs and encouraged you to heed them—along with any other symptoms you suspect spell trouble—I could technically end this chapter right here. But I know better. Simply having information about what might be a red alert doesn't always push people to act. Here's a perfect example. My husband, a doctor who is an infectious disease specialist, once insisted that an infection in his leg was not a problem. I had to plead with him to let me take him to the emergency room! If a doctor can deny what is obvious, you can, too—and probably do. It's human nature not to want to face the fact that something is wrong with you. Magical thinking takes over, as in "If I ignore this, it will just go away. Anyway, I don't have time to be laid up right now, so this can't be happening." Jenny, a forty-year-old wife and mother who almost let denial kill her, talks about how her mind worked on the night she was infected with a virulent combination of the staph and strep bacteria:

"It was my daughter Sarah's tenth birthday and she had invited ten of her friends for a Friday night sleep-over. The plan was to let the girls sleep late the next day, since they would obviously be up giggling until all hours. I was going to make a pancake brunch after they woke up, and then drive them to the beach in our new van. Sarah was so excited she could hardly stand it and I wanted everything to be perfect for her. I'm a lawyer so sometimes I have to work long hours. That's why whenever I get the chance, I really go all out for Sarah. Maybe it's guilt or maybe it's just that I wish I could be in two places at once and not miss so much of her growing up. Whatever it is, I get really intense about stuff like the plans for that birthday weekend.

"Anyway, by about eleven P.M. the girls were all settled in their sleeping bags in the family room watching a video. My husband was already asleep. I was just getting around to looking at the mail. I tore open an envelope and happened to get a paper cut on my right thumb. It started to bleed a little so I sucked on it. When I finished with the mail, I went to bed.

"At three A.M., I woke up with a terrible, throbbing pain in my thumb. I turned on my little reading lamp. My thumb was all purple and swollen. My first reaction was annoyance. I had forgotten about the paper cut and just assumed that I had somehow banged my thumb in my sleep. Why would something so stupid have to happen on a weekend when I was so busy? I got up to go put some ice on my thumb. The family room is adjacent to the kitchen, and Sarah came in to get a drink of water. When she saw my thumb, her eyes got really big, and she said, 'Mommy! What happened?' But I just shrugged and told her it was a little bruise.

"By six A.M., after taking three Advil, I was still wide awake. I decided I might as well make the pancake batter.

About eight A.M., my husband came down for his morning coffee. He looked at my thumb and said, 'What the hell is that?' I mumbled something about being a klutz even in my sleep. But he wasn't buying it. He insisted that I call my doctor right away. I said it could wait until Monday. He said, 'So why are you dancing around like that and gritting your teeth?' Then he picked up the phone and dialed the doctor himself.

"To make a long story short, I had a contracted a serious infection in the thumb, apparently from germs in my own saliva. Because I had let it go for hours, a potentially lethal blood poisoning called septicemia had developed. I ended up in the hospital. When the crisis had passed, the doctor asked me why I had waited so many hours before reporting something so clearly out of the ordinary and painful. I just shrugged. I was too embarrassed to say that I had been planning to drive my daughter and her friends to the beach and didn't want to be interrupted. It seemed so ridiculous in retrospect. But that is how my mind was working at the time. I like to think I'm pretty smart, but I had behaved like a total fool."

Jenny shouldn't be so hard on herself. As I've said, denial is all but universal. But you *can* conquer it. Here's how:

Problem: Whether you're faced with an acute symptom such as Jenny's abscessed thumb or a progressive one like a breast lump, there's a tendency to get caught in the trap of telling yourself "this isn't a good time for me to be sick." There's never a good time. Either your desk is piled with work that you were hoping to finish before the boss found out how far behind you had gotten, or your child's school play is the next day, or it's Christmas Eve, or your long-awaited vacation with the nonrefundable airline tickets is at hand, or . . . you get the idea. Dwelling on how there is no way you can be having appendicitis or a heart attack or a systemic reaction to a bee sting at this particular moment will jam your health radar. You'll miss the signals and put yourself in danger—maybe grave danger.

Solution: Get off the hamster wheel of negative thinking. Start by making actual plans for how you would manage if you found out you really were going to be out of commission for days, weeks, or months. Yes, you are unique and invaluable, but you are not indispensable at the expense of your health. Could a trusted colleague at the office go through the pile of work on your desk and minimize it enough so that the boss wouldn't think you've been slacking? Could someone videotape the school play for you? Could you send flowers to your budding thespian with a note saying how proud you are? Could your sister have your husband and kids over for Christmas dinner if you end up in the hospital? Can you change those airline tickets to a later date by paying a fairly nominal fee? The answer is almost always affirmative to each of the above. And once you've reassured yourself that people will cover for you in an emergency or that you can make contingency plans, you can let down your defenses. You can admit that, yes, you're doubled over in excruciating pain and it's no joke. Or if your symptoms don't constitute an emergency but they've been going on for some time, acknowledge that and say it out loud. You've moved from "This can't be happening!" to "This is happening, and I'm not thrilled, but I can handle it."

Problem: You engage in the magical thinking I mentioned earlier: "This will go away if I just wait awhile. In fact, I think I'm feeling better than I did a minute ago (or yesterday, or last week)." What's happening here is that you're relying on past experience. You've always gotten better sooner or later until now. Why would this situation be any different? Surely, as the old chestnut goes, this, too, shall pass.

Solution: Write down your symptoms. Pick up a pen or go to your computer and make a note such as "The right side of my head feels like it's going to explode" or "I have a mole on my chest that keeps getting bigger." Now read the note out loud to yourself. Whether this is an emergency situation or a progressive problem, the written statement will jolt you into accepting the fact that something is definitely awry. Incidentally, this exercise may be harder than you think. However, the more you resist writing down the symptom, the more likely it is that you are very worried. This is a kind of litmus test for denial. You don't want to face what's happening so you certainly don't want to see it in black-and-white. But force yourself. Your health may be at stake.

Problem: You're embarrassed to tell anyone what's going on because you're in public—maybe at work or in a restaurant or on an airplane. After all, from the time you were a little child you've been learning how to be on your best behavior when you're in certain settings. In large measure, that means overriding your body's urges. You stifle a burp, you don't pass gas, you muffle a sneeze, you control a cough, you swallow a yawn, you don't scratch yourself. A natural extension of that training is that you try to conceal anything your body is doing that wouldn't be acceptable in polite company. That stabbing pain in your gut, which could be appendicitis or an ectopic pregnancy, just isn't something you want to announce in the middle of the annual meeting of the board of directors.

Solution: Since this overly civilized reaction could cost you life or limb, correct for it ahead of time by imagining yourself in embarrassing situations. Then diffuse the bomb of false pride by learning to laugh at what's going on. Remember when President Bush threw up on the Emperor of Japan at a state dinner? The unplanned photo op resulted in front-page pictures around the world, plus endless jokes and snickers. Mentally insert yourself into Bush's place in that incident. Go ahead and laugh. Now mentally rehearse some similar scenes, always with you as the hapless protagonist. In so doing, you're preparing yourself to handle with good grace and prudent haste any threat to your well-being that might overtake you in the future.

Problem: You blame yourself, so you want to keep your condition a secret. We've all read and heard so much information on prevention by now that we've come to believe we should have been able to stave off pretty much any disease or disorder just by eating right, exercising regularly, getting enough sleep, quitting smoking, drinking in moderation, lowering stress levels, and so on. Getting sick can feel like a stigma, so you try to keep your condition to yourself.

Solution: Even if you *are* somewhat at fault for whatever ails you, concealing your condition out of shame or embarrassment will only make things worse. Remember, nobody's perfect. So pay attention to your symptoms. Then get thee to the doctor and 'fess up about your two-pack-a-day habit or your penchant for red meat or your couch potato status. Relax. This is about helping you get well. It isn't Judgment Day. Yet. But it could be soon if you keep putting off getting a diagnosis and treatment. Believe me, you won't be the first person your doctor has seen who has some bad health habits. The doc may even have a few of his own!

Problem: Even if you confide in someone close to you or if someone notices that you're in pain although you're trying to hide it, you don't believe the person's feedback about the possible urgency of your complaint. Jenny, for example, shut out the shocked reaction of her daughter when Sarah saw the abscessed thumb. Jenny also played down her pain when her husband pressed her. This is very common because none of us wants to worry those we love. We want to be strong for them, not vulnerable—and certainly not a burden. Consequently, we turn away from them just when we need them most.

Solution: Flip the scenario around in your head so that your husband (son, mother, maiden aunt) is the one with the worrisome symptom and you are the one trying to get through to that person. In this role, you want to be needed and heeded. You want to help. And you feel angry at this person for being so stubborn. After all, if the worst should happen, you'd be the one left to grieve. Now, do 180 degrees back to reality. You're the one who's being stubborn. You're the one who's taking a chance on your own life while your nearest and dearest is powerless to help.

So stop insisting you're just fine. Be grateful people care and that you don't have to go it alone. Let somebody be what I call your "health buddy." Whoever you pick will serve as a confidant and a coach who encourages you to do what you should to take care of yourself. If you have written about your problem, let your health buddy read your "confession." This person can also come with you to the hospital or to office visits—a boon when you're too sick or frightened to speak for yourself. And when the crisis has passed, the two of you can team up to reach health goals such as losing weight, sticking with an exercise regimen, or quitting smoking. Misery and good intentions both love company!

YES, IT CAN HAPPEN TO YOU

As we have just seen, denial is a psychological coping mechanism which gives you a specious sense of well-being when you're confronted with actual symptoms, whether acute or persistent. But there's a cousin of denial which can also put your health in jeopardy. It comes into play when you have no symptoms and feel just fine. I call it "risk blindness." Let's say your father died of heart disease in his fifties. You are approaching the Big Five-Oh. You've put on a few pounds since you were at your fighting weight in college, and your desk job is so demanding that there's no time to go to the gym. You know you should quit smoking, but you can't concentrate on those piles of paperwork without puffing away. All of this adds up to a heart attack waiting to happen, but you don't think it can happen to you. You're not alone. That sense of being invincible is just about universal, and it's good, in that it keeps us from being chronic worrywarts. We get up every morning and go about our business feeling pretty darn sure we're not going to come down with a horrible illness or get hit by lightning or slip and break a leg. However, the innate panic protection turns against you when you have good reason to expect you might succumb to any given disease, but you ignore that probability and go on pushing your luck.

A perfect example of risk blindness is the case of TV talk show host Regis Philbin. Speaking to a reporter for *Reader's Digest*, he said: "The first time I felt chest pains was early in 1993. They would come and go, so like an idiot I never went to a doctor. My father died in his mid-sixties of heart disease, but I thought it couldn't happen to me." Regis, who was fifty-nine in 1993, went on to describe a subsequent heart attack and angioplasty, and mentioned the fact that his cholesterol level remained at a precariously high 300. Then he talked about the day he had his second attack. "I was scheduled to do a high-wire act with the circus that was in town, and I went ahead with the stunt. I know it was crazy. The minute I got down off the wire, I said to Gelman, my producer, 'Drive me to the hospital.'" Regis went on to say they did an atherectomy, a "Roto-Rooter" to break up the clog, and added: "Then I got really serious about my diet and exercise. . . . I tell people that even with the medication, I have to work out and eat right. And to cope with stress, I listen to Dean Martin. Dealing with Kathie Lee and Gelman every day, I have to have a way to calm myself down! It must be working because it's been over five years since the last heart scare and I've never felt better."

Regis got not one but two extra chances to save his own life. However, if *you* suspect you have any risk factors for a disease, particularly a family history, *don't gamble.* Ask your doctor to go over your health profile with you while you're still feeling great, and then do everything you can to outsmart your genes.

HOW YOUR HEALTH RADAR CAN WORK FOR THOSE YOU LOVE

Until now, we've been talking about how to tap into your instincts about your own health. But you know deep inside that you have a sixth sense about your family's health as well. If the baby's crying sounds different and distressing, trust your fears and call the doctor. If your wife or husband has chest pains and the emergency room personnel say it's nothing, don't accept that conclusion if your gut says it's the wrong diagnosis. I testified for the prosecution in a malpractice case like this in which a man had subsequently died. At the deposition the wife said she didn't argue or get a second opinion because she thought the doctor knew better than she did. I couldn't help but flinch when I heard that. Talk about suffering from the White Coat Syndrome! Respect for authority and expertise is one thing, but to place all the accountability for decision making in the doctor's hands is a terrifying prospect. Doctors are only human. Doctors are often overburdened. Doctors can be sleep-deprived. Blind faith in everything a doctor says about the condition of those you love amounts to abdicating all responsibility for their welfare. You don't want that and neither does your doctor. So let yourself believe that you almost always know best when it comes to your children, your spouse, your aging parents, anyone close to you. Then act on their behalf when you feel they're not getting the attention they need—or for that matter, when you feel they are being given too many tests or too much medication. Have the courage to ask questions when your instincts tell you something may not be right.

—⎷⟋—

As an ancient proverb puts it, "A journey of a thousand miles begins with a single step." Congratulations. You have taken the first step in the journey toward saving your own life. You now know that your doctor needs your expertise as much as you need hers. You also know that you, *and only you*, can say where it hurts and how much and when. Most important, you know that without your input, your doctor will have a much tougher time figuring out *why* it hurts.

You're ready to take the next step. It is at the very core of my philosophy and my plan for teaching you how to save your own life. This key step moves out of the realm of introspection and into the concrete world of your medical records. When you finish Step 2, you will have in your own hands the history of your health—and with it, the power to

Step 1: Trusting Yourself as the Real Expert About Your Health

protect yourself from clerical or computer errors, prevent misdiagnoses, and make certain that everyone involved in your care is fully informed. That kind of power, in an era of ever-increasing depersonalization and fragmentation in our health care system, is nothing short of revolutionary. Follow me . . .

Step 2 Collecting and Studying Copies of Your Medical Records

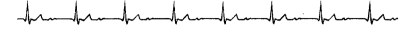

"Ethically and legally, you are entitled to the information in your records."
—American College of Physicians' Code of Ethics

By the time a forty-something woman I'll call Louise arrived at the hospital in response to a frantic call from her mother, her father's breath was coming in short gasps. The doctor on duty told Louise that her father, a seventy-three-year-old we'll call Jim, had a potentially lethal arrhythmia which can be caused by a toxic reaction to the drug digitalis. But since Jim wasn't on that medication, his condition was a mystery.

"He is taking digitalis!" Louise said. The doctor shook his head. Louise's mother had brought a brown bag full of Jim's medications and there was no digitalis in it. Louise insisted that her mother had simply missed that one crucial bottle in her haste to get Jim to the emergency room. She asked the doctor to call the office of the group practice where Jim's medical records were kept. Unfortunately, it was past 6:00 P.M. and the offices were closed. Jim's life hung in the balance, and there was no way short of driving back to the house to look for the bottle of pills to verify that he was on them.

Before I finish this story, I'm going to tell you Louise's real name: Marie Savard, M.D. I was the frightened and helpless daughter in the above scenario. The incident took place in

1998 after I had been a physician for over two decades and a nurse before that. Yet my expertise was all but useless without access to my father's medical records. The good news is that the emergency room personnel started treatment based on the assumption that digitalis was the culprit. My father, John Savard, pulled through. Further good news is that he now carries a complete list of medications and doses in his wallet, and he has collected all his records from various doctors and facilities.

You should, too. The incident involving my father's arrhythmia underscores one important reason. The days when a family doctor had all your information in a manila folder, at the ready day and night, are long gone. In all likelihood your records exist piecemeal in an array of offices, computers, laboratories, and on microfilm at one or more hospitals. If you've moved around a lot, it's a pretty sure bet your records didn't follow you. To be safe, you need to locate as many of them as possible and keep a set of copies where you can get at it anytime you want.

I know that the idea of figuring out where the paperwork is and trying to collect it—much less understand it—sounds overwhelming, but in the end, you'll be glad you made the effort. That's because even though we talk about the health care "system" in this country, there's nothing systematic about it anymore. There are now no clear lines of communication among the professionals who are trying their best to work within it. As my mother would say, the left hand doesn't know what the right hand is doing. That situation probably isn't going to change anytime soon. Plenty of critics have written reams of words railing against the deficiencies of the health care system, and reformers including Hillary Rodham Clinton have struggled to find ways to fix this mess. But so far, nothing has worked. I believe the solution is a grassroots effort, with each of us taking medical matters literally into our own hands.

I hope you won't wait until a crisis occurs to try to cobble together the information that could save your life. You're better off starting now. The last thing you need when you're sick and frightened is to have to think straight enough to remember where your old mammograms might be or what the names of all your medications are. Far better to take the time and trouble to get your medical affairs in order right away and keep them up to date from now on. Consider this a kind of insurance policy that is guaranteed to pay out. After all, you fork over plenty for protection against such things as fire and natural disasters and theft which may well never happen. Why not spend a nominal amount of money and a little of your time to protect yourself against the very real possibility of medical mishaps?

Another reason for gathering your records is that you may find errors which could cost you insurance coverage, employment, or—in the case of allergic reactions—your life. In this electronic age, a lot of people are looking at your files. Some or all of your data are almost certainly in the computers of your insurance company and may even have found their way to a central data bank called the Medical Information Bureau. This organization identifies high-risk patients for insurers, but reportedly some 600,000 of the MIB files contain information that is inappropriate or just plain wrong. You wouldn't necessarily want a prospective boss to know that you're a recovering cocaine addict, and you certainly wouldn't want her to think you have Alzheimer's if you don't.

That's not all. Even though your records shouldn't be released or transferred without your signature, health information often beams through cyberspace unchecked. It then lands in the databases of pharmacies, researchers, and direct marketing companies without your being aware of what happened. Privacy rules proposed by the federal government may not adequately protect your information. You're better off learning exactly what is in your records, and making sure mistakes are corrected. Otherwise, this is clearly an Orwellian situation with Big Brother knowing more about your most personal information than you do.

Finally, if you don't collect your records, they could lawfully be destroyed after two to seven years by the people and facilities who own them. Without a doubt, getting your hands on your records and those of your family as soon as you can is the only way to have both power and peace of mind when it comes to your health care.

HOW TO GET THE JOB DONE

You may have been tempted to delegate the job to one of the computer- or Web-based services that have been cropping up. On closer look, these high-tech versions neither work as well nor cover as many bases as a hard copy system does. One Web company makes this enticing statement: "Imagine the ability to harness the power of the Internet and have all your vital medical history maintained for a small fee in one convenient place in cyberspace." However, the pitch quickly adds these disclaimers: "[We] do not assume responsibility in the event of a technical error. . . .We make great efforts to ensure confidentiality, but the final responsibility for privacy rests with the subscriber. . . .We take no responsibility for the validity or accuracy of the medical information. . . . Under ideal circumstances medical information will be available 24 hours a day, 7 days a week, 365 days a year."

Uh, okay. So you're injured on the interstate miles from home and the computer is down. So much for "ideal circumstances." Not only that, but the information this company stores in cyberspace is just data entry, not original records. I know from experience that copies of original records are the only source of all the data doctors need. The reports use language which telegraphs information to your doctors in a format with which they're comfortable and often contain fine points which could be significant to you. In an emergency, even if all you had on your person was a list of medications and allergies but no documents, someone back home could fax copies of your actual records if that proved necessary. So save the $35 setup fee, the $29 quarterly maintenance, and the $10 for every update which you'd have to spend for the Internet record-keeping service. Doing it yourself is cheaper and far more effective. Similarly, don't rely solely on the new "smart cards" which allow pharmacists and physicians to get your medical history with one swipe through a reader. They sound good, but they'll never be a substitute for your actual detailed documents. Besides, *you* don't have a reader and thus you're left out of the loop, with everyone but you seeing what's on your card.

A better strategy by far is to compile a complete medical history, including copies of your test results, doctors' and hospitals' summaries, emergency room summaries, immunization records, and radiology reports—all of which you are legally entitled to have. In some states, there are laws spelling out patients' rights to their health information. Other states lack such laws. However, there is no state that has a law saying you *can't* have your records. The original documents are owned variously by health care providers, facilities, and insurers, but you can get photocopies. Note: You can also get copies of the records of your minor children. If you are responsible for anyone else—an aging parent, a developmentally delayed sibling, a grandchild, an unrelated child whom you have taken into your home—you must get legal power of attorney in order to access the person's medical records—or for that matter, to get medical help for the person.

DATA COLLECTION 101

Before you attempt to find old medical records, start your collection the easy way. Beginning with your next office visit, request your results and summaries. Give your doctor a self-addressed, stamped envelope and a sticky note with the current date, the records you want sent to you, your name in block letters, your signature, and your date of birth. He can then put the sticky note as a flag on your chart to remind him to follow through. Make a couple of sticky notes for yourself and put them wherever they'll jog your memory—as a flag in your daily agenda, on the refrigerator, or on your calendar. If you don't receive your results within three weeks, make a follow-up phone call.

But I can almost hear you saying that you're worried that asking for your records might antagonize your doctor. To be honest, that's not an unfounded fear. Historically, the two reasons a patient might ask for her records were because she was going to switch doctors or because she wanted to get a second opinion. The first is obviously not a vote of confidence if the choice is the patient's. And even if she's forced to make a change because of a new health plan, the doctor won't be happy about losing her business. Also, while a second opinion is a good idea in the abstract, it, too, implies a lack of trust when you come right down to it. Your doctor is only human, and knowing that you are questioning his judgment can create a rift in your relationship with him.

This is not to say that you shouldn't change doctors or get

a second opinion when you feel the need. Just make certain your doctor understands that your motive right now is simply to get a set of records for yourself so you can work as a team with him and ultimately reduce the risk of malpractice suits. That last point matters a lot. He may have encountered other people who have taken the adversarial stance espoused by some patients' rights activists. They tend to behave as though the issue of patient-held records is an us-against-them battle with the medical establishment. I'm a well-known patients' rights champion myself, but my view is that we're all in this together. When you have access to your own records and come to office visits with a reasonably complete set, it helps your doctor do a better job.

ON THE PAPER TRAIL

When you decide to locate your existing records, work in reverse chronological order. What I mean is that you shouldn't let yourself get stymied by the potentially impossible quest for long-lost records. Track down relatively current records first. First, let all your doctors and practitioners know what you're trying to accomplish by writing a brief, courteous letter to each person who might have what you need. Let's have a look at where your records might be.

I. Your family doctor (and gynecologist) should have the following:

1) Progress notes including a running record of your height, weight, and blood pressure. (The handwritten notes are not particularly helpful, so don't request them.)

2) Typed summaries dictated by specialists you've seen such as cardiologists and urologists.

3) Discharge summaries from hospital stays and the emergency room.

4) Results of all blood work and urinalyses.

5) Pathology reports (Pap smears, biopsies).

6) Radiologists' reports (chest X-rays, mammograms, DEXA scans). (While you're at it, you might consider getting the actual X-rays along with the reports. In theory, if you move and get your next X-rays done elsewhere, the two radiology departments will communicate so that the new radiologist can compare your baseline with the current results. However, in practice that doesn't always happen. Nobody cares as much as you do about your films, so put yourself in a position to hand-deliver them if necessary.)

7) Results of heart testing (EKGs, cardiac stress tests, cardiac echoes).

8) Results of screening and diagnostic tests (sigmoidoscopies, colonoscopies).

9) Your doctor may also have your immunization history. If not, blood tests can determine which antibodies you have if that ever becomes important.

II. In the event that your family doctor does not have consultation reports, which should have been sent to him by specialists, contact the specialists directly. Also, if you regularly see a specialist such as a cardiologist, make a habit of getting your results on an ongoing basis just as you do when you visit your family doctor or gynecologist.

III. In the event that your family doctor does not have hospital discharge summaries, contact the medical records department at the hospital and specifically request the summary. Otherwise you may get (and be charged for) the whole file, which will be redundant and probably include scribbled notes you would have trouble reading.

IV. In the event that your family doctor does not have laboratory results (Pap smears, biopsies) or radiologists' X-ray reports (chest, mammogram, DEXA scans), you can try contacting the lab or the hospital radiology department. This may or may not work, but it's worth a try. You have probably heard that a good ploy for getting the hospital to release your records is to have a doctor friend request them for you, even though your signature is what's required to get them. Unfortunately, this is often true. But I'm against game playing, which only perpetuates the model of the powerless patient. There is strength in numbers and if we all start now to ask for what is rightfully ours, giving patients copies of their records will become commonplace.

V. Contact complementary care clinicians (acupuncturists, physical therapists, chiropractors), as well as eye care specialists, pharmacists, and dentists.

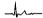

Be aware of the fact that while your doctor keeps your records on file, she may no longer own them. Records are often the property of a hospital or health care system.

When you have made a list of each person and place you're going to contact, make a log to keep track of responses. Jot down next to each entry the date you send your request. Also write the date if you make follow-up attempts by mail or phone. Finally, fill in dates as you receive documents.

Be sure to give your date of birth in all correspondence about your medical records. That's the information that will be used to locate your files, particularly if your records turn out to be in a hospital system. You can send a letter with a self-addressed stamped envelope included, or you can request that your records be faxed to you. (Note: If you have a thermal paper fax machine, your copies may fade over time.) In any case, you should send a check to cover the cost of copying your records. I'd offer from $5 to $15 depending on how many records you're requesting. Again, be specific or you may get a sheaf of useless, scribbled notes along with the typed reports and summaries you're after. Whether or not your doctor accepts the money, she'll appreciate the offer. In a sense, it's the thought that counts here. Yet even if your checks do get cashed, that will be money well spent to get records that could save your life, especially in an emergency.

But what if you don't get your records in spite of the pleasant tone of your letter? I'd give the doctor or facility three weeks to act on your request, and then I'd place a follow-up phone call. You will probably feel annoyed, but avoid being confrontational. You may know the receptionist or office manager, and she may remember who you are from past visits. But give her the benefit of the doubt and say something such as:

> "Good morning. This is Jane Doe, one of Dr. Smith's patients. I'm calling to follow up on a letter I sent about three weeks ago asking for copies of my medical records. I know you're busy and maybe just haven't gotten around to taking care of my request, but I thought I'd better check."

If she says she did indeed get your letter and that she's sorry about the delay but will get to it soon, then you're in business. However, if she tells you that it's not the doctor's policy to send patients copies of their records, don't let yourself be intimidated. There's no need to be rude or antagonistic—which, oddly, is what some patients' rights advocates advise—but do be politely persistent. Even in the case of impersonal institutions, that approach almost always works eventually. Save in-your-face tactics as an absolute last resort. I'd suggest writing an amicable but firm second letter, as follows:

JANE DOE
123 Main Street
Hometown, USA 45678

July 28, 2000

Joseph Smith, M.D.
910 Any Avenue, Suite 11
Hometown, USA 45678

Dear Dr. Smith:

When I spoke with Katrina on the phone this morning, she told me that you are not prepared to honor my request for copies of my medical records because it's not your policy to let patients have access to their charts.

In fact, while you own the documents, the information belongs to me. There is a law in this state which makes that clear. [Or: There is no law in this state preventing patients from obtaining their records.] Again, I am asking for the copies only in order to safeguard against loss and errors, and to allow me to participate more fully in my care.

I appreciate your consideration of this matter, and I look forward to receiving my records shortly. I am enclosing another stamped self-addressed envelope for your convenience.

Sincerely,

Jane Doe
DOB: March 21, 1946

Step 2: Collecting and Studying Copies of Your Medical Records

If you want to find out what your local law is, send $10 to Public Citizen Publications Department, 1600 20th Street NW, Washington, DC 20009-1001 for a state-by-state guide called "Medical Records: Getting Yours," by Bruce Samuels and Sidney M. Wolfe. However, all you really need to know is that you have a right to your records, no matter where you live. When you make your doctor aware of that, he'll almost certainly give you what is legally yours.

FILLING IN THE GAPS

After you have finished collecting your recent records, you can begin to think back to the older ones. However, if you can't locate them or if they have been destroyed, don't lose sleep over it. In the case of immunizations, depending on your age you either had the shots or had the childhood diseases. A blood test will verify that you have the antibodies should that ever become absolutely necessary in order for you to get a job dealing with young children such as teaching or camp counseling. And you can make up for any other lost records by writing down your illnesses, surgeries, hospitalizations, and chronic medical conditions from childhood on. Date your entries in chronological order, giving approximate times if you can't remember whether your mother said you had viral pneumonia at the age of two or three. Beyond that, you can write your own recollection of the knee surgery you had after getting clipped playing football in high school, or the emergency dental work you had done in Paris during your junior year abroad. Just about any information could be important. At the very least, it will save the time and expense of replicating tests. For example, if you have a benign heart condition, there's no need for every practitioner to discover that all over again. My rule of thumb is: When in doubt, write it down.

Also, women should write their menstrual history. Include your menarche (the date of your first period), any events such as amenorrhea (missed periods when you're not pregnant or menopausal) or PMS, plus infertility problems and treatments, pregnancies, miscarriages, details of giving birth (vaginal, breach, cesarean), and menopause. You can leave out abortions if you don't want to disclose that information, but I'd mention it to your gynecologist if there were any complications.

There may be other information which you wouldn't want potential employers to see, such as a history of emotional or psychiatric problems, an HIV positive status, or your sexual orientation. There's no need to write down that information unless you're taking medication. Adverse drug interactions must be avoided at all cost. Also, if you smoke, your doctor absolutely needs to know that.

Speaking of drugs, list any side effects you've experienced. Some may simply be unpleasant, such as an upset stomach from a cholesterol-lowering drug. Others may be life-threatening, such as going into shock after taking penicillin. Still others fall somewhere in between, like staying awake all night if you take the antihistamine Benadryl or having pain get worse instead of better if you take codeine. The idea is to make sure no one prescribes a medication that you already know causes problems for you.

If you have other serious allergies such as a systemic reaction to bee stings, or a life-threatening reaction to seafood or to eating nuts, or severe asthma episodes when you're around cats, write that down. Also, list all your medications. Make a note of dosages, directions, the dates you started and stopped taking each medication and why, the results, and the reason you changed doses if you did so.

Go as far back as you can remember, since one reason for

this list is to let current and future doctors know what did and didn't work for you in the past. For example, if you had recurring bouts of the urinary tract infection called cystitis fifteen years ago and a sulfa drug cleared it up with no notable side effects, that's useful information. Also, writing down from now on the dates you start and stop a drug will help your doctor track your health patterns and adjust your treatment. If you have migraines, your doctor may work out a prevention therapy instead of continuing to treat each new episode. Or if you've taken antibiotics for upper respiratory problems several times in one year, that could tip him off to look for reasons you're sick so often.

As you make your medication list, remember that a drug is a drug whether it's an aspirin, a vitamin, an extract of ginkgo root, or a pill your doctor prescribed to lower your cholesterol. Withholding any information from your health care providers is risky business. Yet a study by the Mayo Clinic showed that over half of the respondents failed to report the use of herbs and over-the-counter drugs.

However, when it comes to illegal recreational drugs and alcohol overuse, confidentiality is a legitimate concern. You certainly need to get help if you have problems in these areas, but you may decide that it's not prudent to put the information in writing and risk having it fall into the wrong hands.

CARRY A LIFESAVER IN YOUR WALLET

Make a personal health information list to carry with you all the time. Tuck it in your wallet right next to your insurance card. Also, give a copy to each of your health care providers. Include the following information: name; date of birth; address; phone; e-mail address; serious adverse reactions to drugs, bee stings, food, X-ray "contrast dyes"; medical conditions (e.g., hypertension, diabetes, osteoporosis, contact lenses, false teeth, a heart murmur that warrants antibiotics before surgery, and any major surgery you've had performed); an up-to-date list of medications, including dose and directions; significant family conditions (early heart disease, diabetes, breast cancer, colon cancer, prostate cancer, and so on); date of last immunization for tetanus/diphtheria, pneumonia, and flu; physician's name, address, and phone number; emergency contact; living will information; durable power of attorney. Notice that I didn't ask you to list your blood type. That's because it's not as important as you probably think it is. Should you need a transfusion, you would be stabilized with fluids while a compatibility check took place. No one would rely on what blood type you had written on your sheet, but put it down if you like.

Ask your doctor to review your health information to make sure it is thorough and accurate. True, that sounds like a bit of an imposition, but any good doctor will help you out.

GET YOUR REPORTS AND RESULTS FROM HERE ON

Don't stop now. Get the results of every test and procedure as they occur in the future. Let your doctor know that you won't make a nuisance of yourself with your requests, and that you'll make things easy for him by handing the office manager a self-addressed stamped envelope with a note giving the current date, the records you want sent to you, your name in block letters, your signature, and your date of birth.

The reason you need to ask for your results may surprise you. Like most people, you have probably thought that no news is good news when it comes to the results of your Pap test or your colonoscopy or your EKG. I'm going to make you privy to a medical insider's secret: No news may be bad news. A recent study in the *Archives of Internal Medicine* has shown that at least 30 percent of physicians do not have a tracking system to alert patients of abnormal test results. You may assume that everything is fine if you don't hear anything, but the truth may very well be that your results were misinterpreted, filed in someone else's folder, or just plain lost. Especially in a large practice, with doctors being rushed to see one case after another and clerical help working with very little supervision, mistakes do happen.

A case in point is Susan Henley. When she switched to a new managed care plan, she was asked to fill out and send in a questionnaire concerning her risks for breast cancer. By return mail, she was advised that because she was forty-eight, postmenopausal, and had a maternal aunt who had the disease, a mammogram was in order. Susan had the test done, and was told she was fine. A month later, she went to her doctor for a routine physical. He had the results of the mammogram in the form of a typed letter in her folder. Glancing at it briefly, he said that indeed everything was fine. He then did a breast exam, and said that was normal as well. No follow-up was recommended.

In fact, the results of Susan's mammogram were somewhat abnormal, revealing asymmetry in the form of a denser area of tissue in the right outer breast. While no specific lump or areas of calcification were seen, the results suggested that further evaluation was necessary. But Susan had no way of knowing that because she never asked to read the actual report herself.

During the ensuing six months, Susan developed an area of fullness and discomfort in the right outer area of her breast, but she ignored it because she was reassured by what she had been told about her mammogram. She let a year and a half go by before telling her doctor that the area of her breast was changing. At that point, a biopsy was done and advanced cancer was diagnosed.

Had Susan requested her test results and studied the written report of the mammogram herself, she would have seen the reference to the asymmetry and she could have brought it to her doctor's attention or asked for a second opinion from a doctor who might pay more attention to her case. She could have gotten an earlier diagnosis and a much better prognosis—perhaps treatment with a simple lumpectomy and a complete cure. As it was, Susan needed a mastectomy, chemotherapy, and radiation. I wish I could tell you that she survived, but she didn't. There is no clearer example than this one of how collecting and studying your own medical records really can save your life.

HOW TO READ YOUR OWN RECORDS

Susan's story also demonstrates that you don't need to worry about trying to decipher your records. For the most part the results are in plain English. Surely Susan would have understood "asymmetry in the form of a denser area of tissue in the right outer breast" and been rightfully concerned. Similarly, "suspicious" means exactly what it says. So does "inadequate." Just use common sense, and ask questions about anything that sets off a warning bell. Of course, the reports may contain some medical terminology you won't understand. Susan's had a section that said "clinical correlation is necessary," a commonly used phrase that is probably not immediately comprehensible to you as a lay person. It means that a radiologist was looking at a film out of context, and that the doctor needed to take into consideration the patient's history and physical examination. Unfortunately, this hedge which protects the radiologist is employed so often that doctors tend to glaze over it. But if you had ever seen that on your own chart and not understood it, you could have gotten the translation from your doctor and asked to have the correlation done. To let your doctor know how this would work, try saying something ahead of time such as this:

> "After I get my own copy of the results in the mail, I won't expect you to spend a lot of your valuable time on the phone with me discussing the findings. If I have a quick question, I'll let Katrina know and have her get back to me with your answer. For any major concerns, I'll schedule an office visit."

Another reason that you should study your own results is that you're the one who's going to spend all the time you need to think about them in light of your family history, lifestyle, and risk factors and turn up possible problems. Let's take the example of cholesterol level. Your total might fall in the normal range, but what matters is the breakdown, including the HDL ("good cholesterol") and LDL ("bad cholesterol") levels as well as the ratio of one to the other and to the triglycerides. Studies have shown that in women, the HDL level is a more important predictor of heart disease than the overall cholesterol or the LDL, while for men the LDL level is the key warning sign. Obviously, each patient needs to look at blood test results in context. A forty-year-old woman who smokes and has a total cholesterol level that is normal may believe she's fine when in fact her HDL is at a dangerous low of 30, putting her at considerable risk for heart disease. The solution is for her to look at her results herself, ask what her risk factors are and what those numbers really mean. The same goes for anyone. Once you have the information, figuring out what your level should be is a no-brainer. For example, when it comes to LDL, your goal should be:

* Under 160 if you have no other risk factors for heart disease.

* Under 130 if two or more of the following apply to you: 1) smoking, 2) being overweight, 3) inactivity, 4) diabetes, 5) a systolic blood pressure over 140, 6) a diastolic blood pressure over 90, 7) an HDL under 35, 8) a close female relative who had heart disease before age fifty-five, 9) a close male relative who had heart disease before age forty-five, 10) you are a male over forty-five, 11) you are a female over fifty-five, particularly if you're not taking estrogen.

* Under 100 if you have heart disease.

The numbers for HDL and triglycerides are not as clear-cut. But if your profile shows a pattern of high LDL, low HDL, and low triglycerides, that spells trouble.

Make it your business to learn simple facts like this about all your conditions. I don't mean that you should get obsessive about poring over your results or turn yourself into a nervous wreck trying to figure out everything that could go wrong with you. I simply want you to read your records carefully and make sure you're satisfied that all is well. Then file them where they'll be safe and at your fingertips if you need them down the line.

Now that you've learned how to collect and read your own medical records, I'm going to ask you to take the next step in becoming an informed health care consumer. The time when patients could sit back and expect doctors to be omniscient is a mere memory. Today's physicians can't possibly be up on every new advance and specialty. What's wonderful is that research has yielded breakthroughs in diagnostic techniques and treatment options that can help you live longer and feel better. But the corollary is that you need to learn all you can about your own conditions, diseases, and injuries. This is not as formidable an undertaking as it might sound. In fact, your foray into the field of medicine will demystify aspects of your care that once seemed like scary mumbo jumbo. Turn the page for a guide to gaining the medical knowledge that will let you be confident, aware, and in control.

Step 3 Researching Your Conditions, Diseases, and Injuries

"Because no prescription is more valuable than knowledge."
—C. Everett Koop, M.D.

I began my health care career as a nurse. I soon decided to become a doctor because I felt frustrated by the fact that I didn't have enough power to be as effective as I knew I could be in treating patients. Ironically, in my role as a physician I have come full circle, so that I now believe I have been invested with too much power. The long-standing paradigm of an awestruck patient at the mercy of an all-knowing authority figure in a white coat doesn't work anymore. After all, the word "doctor" comes from the Latin word *docere*, "to teach." As physicians, we are not meant to command blind obedience, but to educate.

Nonetheless, while I once had the luxury of implementing my newfound philosophy by spending as much time as necessary to get my patients involved in their own health issues, the advent of managed care changed that. At one point, when I was in a group practice, I was formally limited to a scant fifteen minutes per patient. Worse yet, studies show that many people get only seven minutes of personal interaction per visit with their doctors.

Yes, this amounts to nothing less than a national disgrace. But I don't want to waste a minute of your time with hand-

44

wringing. Let's just accept the dismal fact that even the best of doctors may not have the time to get deep into the details of your case these days unless you're practically at death's door. In general, doctors try to fix patients who are broken, but not patients who are merely chipped. That's why it's so important for you to study your own medical records and get a working knowledge of your conditions. This is crucial whether you have a life-threatening disease or simply a nuisance ailment that impairs your quality of life. People tend to snap to attention when a health crisis such as cancer strikes, but being well informed is equally vital when you're dealing with less dramatic medical disorders.

A case in point: Maureen, an acquaintance of mine, took her teenage son to their primary care provider for a routine physical. Two weeks later, Maureen received a form in the mail listing the following broad categories: cholesterol profile, sugar, blood chemistry, total blood count, thyroid function, liver function, and urine analysis. All of these were checked off as "normal," just as they had been in previous years. However, because Maureen had heard me talk about the importance of getting copies of original test results, she decided that this time she'd call the office and ask the secretary to fax the actual blood work from the laboratory.

"A lot of the words in the test results were Greek to me," Maureen remembers. "I had no idea what 'creatinine' or 'globulin' meant. But what I did understand were the column headings. One said 'In Range,' another said 'Out of Range,' and then there was 'Reference Range.' I looked at Jeremy's results and saw that his glucose was out of range. I mean, *way* out. His number was 44 and the reference range was 70–115. I thought about calling the doctor to ask for an explanation. But I decided that since he hadn't been concerned enough to check 'abnormal' on the form he sent, he would probably give me the brush-off. So I began doing some research on my own."

What Maureen eventually turned up—and had confirmed by more tests ordered by a physician recommended by a friend—was that Jeremy has chronic low blood sugar. The medical term is hypoglycemia. "He's not going to die from it," Maureen says, sounding admirably well informed and at ease with her topic. "It's not even as big a deal as the opposite problem, which is diabetes. But believe me, it's no small matter. Finding out about this has literally changed Jeremy's life—not to mention mine! The symptoms are fatigue, headaches, irritability, depression, temper outbursts, difficulty making decisions, and lack of motivation. That's quite a list, and it describes Jeremy to a T. To be honest, we had always known that he'd get cranky unless he ate on schedule. He's a basically sweet kid. But from the time he was a little boy, he would do this Jekyll and Hyde number if he got too hungry. He'd be playing nicely in the sandbox at the park and then, wham, he'd burst into tears or push another kid. Then he'd feel terrible and apologize. It was almost like he wasn't himself for a minute there. My solution was to carry snacks all the time. But as he got older and was on his own more, he didn't always do that. Once, he got into a fight at school and he came home absolutely miserable. He said, 'Mom, what is wrong with my brain?'"

Maureen's sleuthing also turned up some frightening statistics showing that hypoglycemics may be prone to aggressive, criminal, and suicidal behavior. "Obviously, no one is as interested in Jeremy's case as he and I are," Maureen says. "The doctor saw a polite, healthy-looking kid and even though Jeremy says he did mention some of his symptoms, we would never have gotten a diagnosis if we hadn't followed through ourselves." The end of this success story:

Maureen got a referral from the second doctor for Jeremy to see a nutritionist. Because Jeremy had a diagnosis from a physician, the insurance company covered the visits. Maureen also bought a low blood sugar cookbook and hooked Jeremy up to a support group online. A year later, he is almost symptom-free and is happier than he's ever been in his life. He's doing well in school, has a girlfriend, and is applying to colleges with an enthusiasm his mother never expected to see. "We could have put him on Prozac," Maureen muses. "And all he needed was the right diet and some support!"

Moral: Whatever is off-kilter, be it of minor or major significance, matters big time to the person who is affected. That's why *you* are the best person to make a concerted effort to find out all there is to know about your own and your family's health problems. Fortunately, in this information age, that is not as tall an order as it may seem. To help you, I'm going to discuss reliable resources, both real and virtual, and steer you clear of those that are less valuable.

THE BOOKS YOUR DOCTOR USES TO LOOK IT UP

There are several lay handbooks out there, most notably the home edition of the *Merck Manual of Medical Information* and *The Johns Hopkins Family Health Book*, but I wouldn't rely solely on those if I were you. They are comprehensive, but the dumbing down often results in entries that are not as in-depth as you need. I honestly believe that there's no reason you can't read the same reference works your doctor reads. As one patient quoted in the *Journal of the American Medical Association* put it: "We have general knowledge about medical things because you see it everywhere—it's all over the news. We are a very informed society." This statement was part of an article celebrating the first anniversary, in May 1999, of the *JAMA*'s monthly "Patient Page," which is designed for doctors to photocopy and leave in their waiting rooms. Focus groups of doctors and patients reported widely divergent views regarding the effectiveness of the page. The physicians thought the page should be brought down to a sixth-grade reading level or lower, that medical terms should be eliminated, and that the size of the type should be made much larger. However, the patients said they had no trouble understanding the page, that they did not want the writing simplified, that they loved reading the actual medical terms, and that they were willing to put up with small type in order to have as much information as possible crammed onto the page in each issue.

I'm sure that like the patients in the *JAMA* focus group, you would rather not have your medical information watered down. That's why I'm sending you straight to the classic texts: *The Merck Manual of Diagnosis and Therapy* and *Harrison's Principles of Internal Medicine*, which is also available on CD-rom. True, some of the lingo might be unfamiliar. But you can always whip out a medical dictionary. Even doctors have to do that from time to time. I use *Mosby's Medical Encyclopedia; Mosby's Pocket Dictionary of Medicine, Nursing and Allied Health;* and *Dorland's Illustrated Medical Dictionary*. If you're only going to buy one, choose *Dorland's*.

Here's an example of why plowing through the standard texts can be more fruitful than using only the books written—as the *Merck* home edition puts it—in "everyday language." When Maureen started her quest for information about Jeremy's hypoglycemia, she first looked in the home *Merck*. She got a fair overview of the disorder along with this advice: "Nondiabetics who are prone to hypoglycemia often can avoid episodes by eating frequent small meals rather than the usual three meals a day." That was all right as far as it went, effectively confirming what Maureen had always known anyway, but she was not satisfied. Even if dietary changes were the whole answer to Jeremy's problem, Maureen yearned to know *why* her son had apparently been born with hypoglycemia. So she bought the seventeenth edition of the version of *Merck* which doctors use. It is, by the way, the centennial edition and comes with a facsimile of the original 1899 volume for those of us who would like to marvel at how very far medicine has come.

In any case, Maureen combed the entry on hypogylcemia in the *Merck* intended for physicians. She found this parenthetical note in a sentence referring to infants and children: "(See also Hypoglycemia in Ch. 260.)" That cross-reference had been omitted in the home version, presumably to avoid overloading lay readers with esoteric bits of information. But when Maureen thumbed her way to Chapter 260, she found a section on hypoglycemia in postmature infants. She was astonished. Jeremy had indeed been born long past Maureen's due date by emergency cesarean section because of fetal distress. Maureen then went back to the home version of *Merck* and looked up postmature infants in the index. Sure enough, the information about hypoglycemia was included, but she wouldn't have known to look for it without a cross-reference. "I like having both the doctors' edition and the home edition," Maureen concludes. "The real one can be hard going, but it has absolutely all the information. I'd recommend starting there, and then if you get stymied you can always go to the lay version for a translation."

Maureen now wishes she had been asking to have the results of Jeremy's blood work from the day he was born.

She has not been able to track down his old records. Without them, the connection between Jeremy's postmature birth and his current condition is hypothetical. But in her own defense, Maureen points out that she had no idea back then that she was entitled to be privy to her own or her family's medical records. "If I had known then what I know now, I would have been reading Jeremy's medical records all along and keeping them on file," she says. "We'd have a history to go on, and we would surely have gotten him to a nutritionist a long time ago."

Yet while Maureen laments not having the early test results, her story proves that late is most definitely better than never when it comes to patient-held medical records. Maureen didn't get clued in to Jeremy's problem until he was almost seventeen years old, but now she's a meticulous record keeper not only for him but for herself and her whole family. She has also become an inveterate medical researcher. "She looks everything up," says Jeremy with an appealing grin. "I call her Dr. Mom. But it's way cool. She ordered a book for me written by a guy who has the same thing I do and that book rocks. I feel better just knowing I'm not a weirdo and that other people have this."

Maureen also did some surfing on the World Wide Web, but before we get into cybermedicine, I have a tip for you about researching medications. Don't bother to buy the *Physician's Desk Reference,* commonly referred to as *PDR.* All it contains is verbatim copies of the package inserts that come with prescription drugs. You can simply read the information that accompanies any drug your doctor prescribes. The manufacturers are required by law to list contraindications and possible side effects. In addition, though, you might want to pick up a copy of *The Essential Guide to Prescription Drugs: Everything You Need to Know for Safe*

Drug Use by James J. Rybacki, Pharm. D., and James W. Long, M.D. Also good are *The Alternative Health and Medicine Encyclopedia*, and *The Nutrition Bible*.

MEDICINE ON THE WEB: A GUIDE FOR CYBERCITIZENS

A recent study showed that 43 percent of Americans now surf the Web for health information. If you're among that number, you have probably already discovered that along with a wealth of useful sites there is also a plethora of cyberquackery. Unlike print media, the Internet allows anyone to "publish" without review or fact checking or standards of any kind.

Another problem is that a random search can waste your time by pointing you to sites that have arcane facts which don't pertain to your situation. You may also wander into sites that are unduly alarming. One of my patients, a fifty-something woman we'll call Peggy, came to me for a second opinion after being diagnosed with hypercalcemia (high blood calcium). Her doctor had ordered a new blood test to be sure that the original reading wasn't a lab error. But when she asked him what the condition might mean, he said, "Let's get the lab work back before you start worrying about that." Frustrated, she went home and typed the word "hypercalcemia" into a search engine on her computer. The first site she happened onto turned out to be advice about dealing with hypercalcemia in iguanas, at reptilian.org. The next place she ended up was a cancer support group containing discussions of hypercalcemia by patients already diagnosed with various malignancies.

That's when she called me in a panic. I calmed her down and explained that while hypercalcemia can be associated with cancer, in asymptomatic cases like hers it is probably something much less serious. I told her to ask for a copy of

51

her blood work and bring it to her office visit with me. Here is yet another instance in which a patient was flabbergasted to hear that she is entitled to her own results. She had already called the first doctor to tell him she was going for a second opinion. She thought that he would automatically send her results to me. What she didn't know is that the doctor is not authorized to release the results without her signature. I would have had no information about Peggy when she arrived if I hadn't prompted her to get her own results. I got into the habit of doing that after I spent one intake interview after another talking with patients about whom I had not a scrap of paperwork.

Peggy did as I asked and by the time she came to me, she was already feeling less terrified. She had seen that her calcium was 10.8, while the reference range for the lab which did her work is 8.1–10.3. She didn't do any more research until after she saw me, but she correctly assumed that an elevation as slight as hers most likely didn't signal disaster. I told her I thought her doctor was going to talk to her about treatment options. The worst-case scenario would be surgical excision of a parathyroid gland and the best-case scenario would be simple medical surveillance. She breathed a huge sigh of relief. I then gave her copies of relevant articles. I also said that since she is obviously interested in researching her condition, she should start by reading the entries on hypercalcemia in *Merck* or *Harrison's* or both. After that, she could venture out into the labyrinthine land of the Internet with refined search terms.

She did what I suggested. First, she tried "hyperparathyroidism" with no results. Then she tried "parathyroid." Bingo! HotBot pointed her to "Parathyroid Disorders and Treatments," an award-winning site with over seventy pages of accessible, reader-friendly text written by leading experts in the field, plus sixty-five illustrations and actual patient X-rays. The site also boasts chat rooms, bulletin boards, an internal search engine, and up-to-the-minute newsletters, as well as a directory of parathyroid specialists across the nation and a directory of support groups. Trust me, not even the best primary care doctor in the world has the time (or interest) to get as conversant with parathyroid problems as Peggy herself has become via that Web site. In the end, Peggy went back to her own doctor, who eventually gave her a diagnosis of hyperparathyroidism. She asked for a referral to a specialist. She brought copies of her test results to the specialist. He ordered a DEXA scan (see page 100), and when Peggy's results came back normal, they decided together on the conservative "watch and wait" option. Peggy has so far avoided surgery and feels great.

You may wonder why I had Peggy use an ordinary search engine instead of going to one of the top-rated medical sites and searching from there. The reason is that the internal databases and search engines at most medical sites may not cover your condition. If you do find what you're looking for, you'll often be led only to scholarly articles or Q&A columns. At best, you'll be redirected to precisely the type of dedicated site or Web ring which Peggy found on her own for parathyroid problems.

I know this from experience. I tried a search for a medical condition, Gilbert's syndrome, a benign congenital disorder in which a person has an elevated bilirubin level. On Thrive.com, one of the best medical sites, I found a fairly good discussion of the topic at "Ask Dr. Bill." But when I went out onto the Web by myself, I found more extensive information. There is an excellent Gilbert's page on the American Liver Foundation site. I also made my way to "Gilbert's Web." This site includes a printable form for patients to carry in order to avoid misdiagnosis of a liver disorder in an emergency situation. It also has a bulletin board. I was interested to see that many people who have Gilbert's syndrome dispute the label "asymptomatic." They have a point. While the syndrome is certainly not dangerous, it can result in mild jaundice or yellowing of the eyes and skin after vomiting or skipping meals, or when the person exercises vigorously or has the flu. I imagine that if you have Gilbert's, jaundice does qualify as a symptom! From my point of view as a doctor, however, I have to admit that if you came in for a visit brandishing printouts of people "discussing" their symptoms on the Internet, I wouldn't take your research all that seriously. My personal purview of the postings on the Gilbert site revealed, along with some sensible stuff, a lot of ranting. Many people claimed to have a host of symptoms which surely had causes other than Gilbert's. Here again, it is the unfiltered nature of a general Web search which makes it simultaneously the route to valuable information and the path to pure hokum. Common sense is your best guide.

Yet while I'm advocating general Web searches instead of going through the medical Web sites—particularly for obscure problems—I'm certainly not dismissing those sites altogether. For one thing, there is great value in the general and news-breaking features of health and medical sites with a magazine format. Because of the instantaneous nature of Web publishing, editors are able to keep you up to the minute. Many of them subscribe to ReutersHealth.com, which means you'll see similar articles at several sites on any given day. (You can visit Reuters yourself, but unless you pay $149 a year, you'll only have access to headlines and abstracts.) One morning, I found articles on the antioxidant properties of apple juice in the *New York Times*, the *Philadelphia Inquirer*, and on a number of health sites including DrKoop.com and AllHealth.com at iVillage on the Web. However, because the e-zines (electronic magazines) are devoted to health issues, the Web articles were more in-depth than the newspaper features. They were also written in the same chummy, we-care-about-you style that makes print magazines so popular. In addition, the e-zines have interactive features such as support group chat rooms and ask-the-expert functions that give them great appeal. Just as you would with print magazines, shop around until you find your favorites from the following list which I recommend to my patients:

AllHealth
http://www.allhealth.com/

This site on the women's network called iVillage is well written and chock-full of great articles, columns, links, and newsbreaks. Joining is free. You'll find a weekly health poll and a host of support groups, including one called "Whine & Cheese." Special sections include among others "Never Say Diet," "Heart Watch" from the publishers of the *New England Journal of Medicine*, "Senior Health," "Alternative Health," "Sexual Health," and "Children's Health." Two recent lead stories were "Kick Butt: Stop Smoking Now with Our 24-Hour Support" and "No Small Change: Find Out About Perimenopause." A feature called "Digital Conscience" lets you pick either "Mom," "a friend named Constance," or a "Coach" to send you weekly encouragement via e-mail to get you to a specified goal such as losing weight. Like all e-zines, this one is sponsored. You'll be encouraged to visit the ads, but that's up to you.

DrKoop.com

http://www.drkoop.com/

The former Surgeon General offers free membership and such departments as "Personal Insurance Center" and "Daily Health with Dr. Nancy Snyderman," a staffed network of interactive communities, healthy recipes, and a service that helps you find "partner" hospitals near you. Be aware that the latter are paid advertisements. There is also information on clinical trials, plus a reasonably extensive internal search engine, an encyclopedia, and health and wellness links.

Health A to Z

http://www.HealthAtoZ.com/

This site offers a calendar feature which will e-mail you reminders about doctor's appointments, prescription refills, and dates when you're due for screening tests. You can also send electronic get-well cards from the site. There are many "supportive communities" including a Night Owls' chat room from 9:00–11:00 P.M. Eastern Standard Time for caregivers of chronically or terminally ill loved ones. A recent lead article had a "life clock" to help you predict how long you'll live, and there is a user-written humor column. "Health Alert" and "In the News" are this site's take on the Reuters releases.

Intelihealth

http://www.intelligenthealth.com/index1.html

This offering was developed by a team of medical and nutraceutical experts. It is directed by physicians and focuses on both traditional medicine and "scientifically based emerging complementary therapies." There is an emphasis on disease prevention, diet, behavior modification, and achieving optimum well-being. When you click on "Health Matters," you'll be directed to internal links for scores of related articles.

Mayo Clinic Health Oasis

http://www.mayohealth.org/

A People's Choice "Webby" award winner in 1999, this site from the renowned clinic has articles originally published in the *Mayo Clinic Health Letter* along with quizzes, headline news, and an array of centers such as "Women's Health," "Men's Health," and "Nutrition." One lead story looked at the issue of marijuana as medicine.

Mediconsult

http://www.mediconsult.com/

Calling itself the "Virtual Medical Center," this zine hosts regularly scheduled live events on such topics as "Living with Lupus," "Living to 100," and "Managing Menopause." Along with the usual array of columns and departments, the site links to such "information partners" as Medizine and PharmInfoNet. Mediconsult subscribes to the Health on the Net (HON) principles, which cover such issues as accuracy of information and confidentiality, and has a legal disclaimer stating that the site is not meant to replace the patient's relationship with his doctor.

OnHealth.com

http://www.onhealth.com/ch1/

A special feature of this site is "OnHealth Shopping," an encrypted cyberstore that accepts your credit information and ships health products, books, and vitamins. "OnHealth Live" invites expert guests to answer users' questions in real time. There are also live Webcasts such as a recent one of actual endometriosis surgery performed at the Stanford University Medical Center. The Webcasts are archived in case you miss a favorite one. Other features: "Daily Briefing," "Today's Health Tip," "Local Health Directory," "Conditions A–Z," and an e-mail newsletter.

ThriveOnline.com
http://www.thriveonline.com/index.html

Billing itself as "The #1 Consumer Health Site," Thrive is stylish, peppy, and full of quick reads about myriad topics. The site has an emphasis on fitness, nutrition, and sex. A resident "sexologist" answers user questions. There's a "Health Library," a "Recipe Finder," and a "Weight Loss Center," plus contests, polls, quizzes, news, and message boards.

WebMD
http://my.webmd.com/index.html

Not as glitzy as some of the other e-zines but packed with information, this entry has a medical encyclopedia, drug reference, self-care advisor, health topics A–Z, breaking medical news, and moderated online chats on topics such as "Dealing with Post Traumatic Stress Disorder" and "Infertility." There is a bookshelf, a library, and a list of communities that serve as online support groups for such diseases as asthma, arthritis, and diabetes.

Beyond that, in spite of what I said about doing your search on your own, you may want to try the following starting points. These are particularly good if you are an Internet "newbie" who is a bit intimidated by the massive and disorganized maze you've just entered.

Healthgate

http://www.healthgate.com/

The mission statement of this for-profit data corporation is as follows: "Our objective is to facilitate improvements in patient care, biomedical research, and education by employing state-of-the-art technology to make information access and coverage both thorough and easy, while maintaining the highest standards of academic and scientific integrity." There is a section for health care professionals and a section for patients. After a four-week free trial, there is a fee for membership.

Medical Matrix

http://www.medmatrix.org

This site is not free. Check for the current fee. Although the site is intended for health care professionals, I doubt that you'll have much trouble understanding the posts. There are thousands of ranked, peer-reviewed, annotated, updated clinical medicine resources. Users can attend symposia via real audio as well as continuing medical education (CME) courses online. There are also links to textbooks, journals, Medline, R_X Assist, a patient education section, and a statistics search.

Medscape

http://www.medscape.com/

Designed for doctors, the site is subtitled "The Online Resource for Better Patient Care." Why not pop in for a visit now and then to see what doctors are reading? Under the head "Clinical Features" are sections on clinical management with "state-of-the-art interactive e-med texts that define the knowledge base and treatment options within each specialty"; a constantly updated list of conferences and symposia;

an ask-the-expert column; links to continuing medical information sites (CME); and a self-assessment feature for physicians. There are also specialty sites (cardiology, oncology, and so forth). Access to over 25,000 full-text journal articles is free, and access to the Dow Jones Interactive Publications Library is on a pay-per-view basis.

Pubmed
http://www.ncbi.nlm.nih.gov/PubMed/

A service of the National Center for Biotechnology Information (NCBI) and the National Library of Medicine (NLM) located at the National Institutes of Health (NIH), this site for professionals uses the Medline database of over nine million articles. Premedline offers abstracts before the full texts are available.

The Best Medical Resources on the Web
http://www.priory.com/other.htm

There is a disclaimer on this site as follows: "PLE Ltd accepts no legal or ethical liability for the contents of websites and resources beyond our space. Sites listed on these pages are listed in good faith following review for quality and apparent validity. Websites change over time and we cannot guarantee the form or content of sites outside our space." That amounts to saying you're not necessarily going to find much reliable stuff by using this gateway, which is by and large correct. For example, if you click on "general medicine," you get a hodgepodge of choices such as "The Aahchoo Directory" and "Tropical Medicine," along with more mainstream places like the Mayo Clinic. Not all listed sites are hot-linked, which means you have to copy down the URLs and type them in yourself. So in spite of the promising title, this site doesn't get my seal of approval.

The Global Health Network

http://www.pitt.edu/HOME/GHNet/GHNet.html

Created at the University of Pittsburgh and sponsored by NASA, this award-winning site is accessible in seven languages and features high-quality information from around the world.

About.com

http://www.about.com

A general portal to the Web with a section on health and fitness, the site has this slogan: "We mine the Web so you don't have to." There are human guides at the ready to help you in real time. When I visited, I chatted with Jennifer. She obliged me by pointing me to my desired topic, placing a "Click Here" button in the dialogue box. Ingenious, and a good place to start if you're a timorous technophobe.

You can also begin at the following sites to find hot links to other sites about your topic:

Mental Health Net

http://mentalhelp.net/

One of the oldest and largest mental health communities online, Mental Health Net combines some of the features of an e-zine (columns, latest headlines, discussions of current news events and research in the field) with the capabilities of a search engine and links to outside sites.

National Institutes of Health

http://www.nih.gov/

This is an exhaustive resource with an internal search engine. For example, typing in "cancer" gets you to thousands of journal articles as well as to the government's Cancernet portal.

Oncolink
http://cancer.med.upenn.edu/

Established in 1992 by the University of Pennsylvania, this is the premier portal for cancer information on the Web. The site has a powerful search engine, a cancer FAQ (frequently asked questions), disease-oriented menus, psychosocial support, personal experiences, cancer screening advice, prevention advice, book reviews, an exhibition of art by people whose lives have been touched by cancer, information on clinical trials, global resources, advice on pain and symptom management, lists of conferences and meetings, and help with financial issues.

Finally, you can find online reference works similar or identical to the books I discussed earlier, as well as online versions of respected medical journals:

Harrison's Online
http://www.harrisonsonline.com/

For $89 a year, you can view on your computer screen the contents of the print version of *Harrison's*, which goes for $99 a copy. Obviously, the online option ends up being by far the most expensive, but the advantage is that it is constantly updated. This is probably more than a lay person needs to spend for that benefit, but the choice is yours.

Merck Manual
http://www.merck.com/pubs/mmanual/

Merck is free online, and organized in an easy-to-access

fashion. Not only the general text but also such specialty editions as "Geriatrics" and "Veterinary Medicine" are posted. This is a gold mine of the very best medical information available—and it's yours for the clicking!

R_xList
http://www.rxlist.com/

Here is your online source for information about prescription drugs, over-the-counter preparations, and alternative/complementary remedies. The site also has patients' personal experiences, a humor column, and a twenty-four-hour-a-day online pharmacy.

The Journal of the American Medical Association
http://www.jama.com

You can read selected articles and editorials, then discuss them in online forums. There is an archive, a patient page, and an impressive stash of peer-reviewed resources on specific conditions. The full text of an interesting article on the quality of medical information on the Web is available. The conclusion: "Many incompletely developed instruments to evaluate health information exist on the Internet. It is unclear, however, whether they should exist in the first place, whether they measure what they claim to measure, or whether they lead to more good than harm." The site is free.

The New England Journal of Medicine
http://www.nejm.org/content/index.asp

You need to subscribe to the print version at $129 a year in order to access full text articles online. However, you can read specially selected articles for free, as well as abstracts of other articles and titles of brief reports and reviews. If you want to read an entire article, report, or review, you can get

reprints by fax or snail mail. Also, all users whether sub-
scribers or not can see "Images in Clinical Medicine,"
"Editorials," "Sounding Board" articles (opinion pieces),
"Correspondence," and "Book Reviews."

A LITTLE KNOWLEDGE DOESN'T HAVE TO BE A DANGEROUS THING

When I talk to doctors about encouraging patients to
research their conditions, I am sometimes met with the concern that we will create a population of the worried well. I
also hear the argument that people will either become confused by medical terminology or thrown off track by erro-
neous or inapplicable information. The story about Peggy
initially getting lost while surfing the uncharted waters of the
Internet and panicking about a benign condition might seem
to corroborate this point of view. But remember that as soon
as I pointed Peggy in the right direction, she became a partner with her doctor. The knowledge she gained allayed her
fears and let her participate in the decision about her care. I
firmly believe that learning about your own symptoms and
problems is good medicine. In Peggy's case, the end result
of seeing for herself the secrets her own blood work
revealed was nothing but positive. Not knowing is simply
never a good idea. Study after study has shown that patients
who feel in control and have an idea of what's going to happen during procedures and treatments can tolerate pain better. They also consistently have far better health outcomes.

Sometimes, even one lone fact about your health can
make all the difference. Here is a chilling example from a
malpractice case in which simply looking at a picture in the
home edition of *Merck* could have saved a young man's life.

Angelo was an immigrant from Italy with a very limited
command of English. Over time, he noticed that the inside

of his right cheek was going numb. He found himself accidentally biting it and not even noticing until he would open his mouth to brush his teeth and see a lesion. He went to a doctor and haltingly explained his problem. The report says he mentioned that his "face felt funny" and that he indicated the right side. If there were ever a case that proves the wisdom of having a health buddy, this is it. Angelo worked at a restaurant and several of his fellow waiters spoke fluent English as well as Italian. He could certainly have used an interpreter!

Not bringing a buddy along was his first mistake. His second was accepting the doctor's diagnosis without question. Angelo was told that he had Bell's palsy, a sudden and benign irritation of the seventh cranial nerve which causes temporary paralysis of facial muscles. Patients sometimes report numbness, but sensations actually remain normal. In other words, a person with Bell's palsy would know it if he bit his cheek. Also, standard practice is to rule out brain tumors when a patient complains of persistent or unexplained facial paralysis. However, Angelo's doctor did not order a CAT scan or an MRI. He sent Angelo home, telling him that the disorder usually disappears in one or two months. If Angelo had known about the home *Merck* and opened it to page 341, he would have seen a drawing of a face with one side of the mouth smiling but the other turning downward, and one eye wide open but the other lid drooping. He would have then looked in the mirror, smiled, and concluded that he didn't have the symptoms that distinguish Bell's palsy from other possible causes of "feeling funny" on one side of the face.

As it was, he went about his business until one day he chomped on his cheek so hard that his pals took him to the emergency room to have the swelling looked at. Six months had gone by and his condition had obviously gotten worse.

But when he told the hospital personnel about his original diagnosis, they accepted that. After all, sometimes Bell's palsy does persist for up to a year. Again, Angelo was sent home and told to wait for the condition to go away. Four months later, his face had swelled so much that he went to an eye, ear, nose, and throat specialist. An MRI revealed a tumor behind his right ear. A biopsy showed that the tumor was malignant. Ten months earlier, it would have been operable and Angelo's prognosis would have been good. But by the time he got his correct diagnosis, it was too late. Angelo died at the age of twenty-five.

His wife sued for malpractice and won, but what a hollow victory. Yes, the doctor should have been more thorough and yes, the emergency room personnel had a duty to reconsider the original diagnosis. But if Angelo had done even one small piece of research, he would almost certainly still be alive. Whether doctors *should* get it right every time is a moot point. So is whether they *could* even if they tried. Mistakes happen, either because of sloppiness or time pressure or lack of up-to-date knowledge or bad guesses. To err is human. In the words of George Bernard Shaw: "As to the honor and conscience of doctors, they have as much as any other class of men, no more and no less."

So don't put your life entirely in your doctor's hands. Instead, collaborate with her. You already know that your instincts are valid, that you need to get your own records, and that you can't afford not to become knowledgeable about what ails you. Let's move right along to Step 4. You'll learn which screening and diagnostic tests and immunizations you need, and when. With this information, you'll be able to ask your doctor to schedule the preventive measures and give you referrals if necessary. (No, she won't necessarily do any of that unless *you* bring up the subject!)

Step 4 Learning Which Immunizations, Exams, and Tests You Need and When

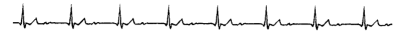

"An ounce of prevention is worth a pound of cure."
—Anonymous

When was your last tetanus shot? When do you need the next one? Are you due for a pneumonia or flu vaccine? A colonoscopy? A screening test for prostate cancer? If you're typical, you're not sure of the answers to those questions. People tend to keep better records of their children's and their pets' inoculations than they do of their own. And while most women know about Pap smears and mammograms, the public's awareness about other screening and diagnostic tests and procedures is not all that high. This fourth step of my guide to saving your own life is meant to remedy that situation. You'll learn how to plot your personal prevention schedule so you can let your doctor know which shots, exams, and tests you need and when. You'll also be able to understand your test results. _

IMMUNIZATIONS YOU NEED

Recommendations for immunizations are fairly clear-cut, although there are exceptions to the rules:

Tetanus/Diphtheria Booster You should get one every ten years. If you can't remember when you had your last shot, have one now and start keeping track from here on. It won't hurt you to have a shot now even if your last one was less than ten years ago. That way, you won't have to ruin a day at the beach by leaving to get a shot if you step on a rusty nail.

Influenza Vaccine (Flu Shot) Because the virus is grown in eggs, don't get this shot if you are allergic to eggs. Otherwise, have it every fall if you're over sixty-five. If you're younger but you have a chronic lung or heart condition, or if you're a health care worker, you should have this shot every fall. Many doctors now recommend yearly flu shots beginning at age fifty.

Pneumococcal (Pneumonia) Vaccine You need this shot once after you turn sixty-five. If you're younger and have special health problems such as lung disease, kidney disease, or any condition which has compromised your immune system, discuss with your doctor whether you should get this shot and whether to repeat it.

Measles/Mumps/Rubella If you were born before 1957, you probably had the diseases and developed natural immunity. A blood test can check for antibodies if you are required to know for sure, such as when you're applying for a health care, teaching, or camp counselor position. All people born after 1957 should have two shots. If you were born before the 1970s, you were probably given your shots when you were too young to develop antibodies. A blood test will confirm this and you can get a booster. Children born after 1970 got their shots at the correct time and don't need boosters. Warning: Pregnant women should *not* get this shot.

Step 4: Learning Which Immunizations, Exams, and Tests You Need

Chicken Pox (Varicella) Most people had this during child-hood and developed antibodies. If you didn't have the disease as a child, you should have two shots one month apart. If you're not sure, a blood test for antibodies will give you the answer. Warning: Pregnant women should *not* get this shot.

Hepatitis B This immunization was not available before the 1980s. It is now automatically given to all newborns and recommended for adolescents who may become sexually active. It is also recommended for health care workers, people who share living quarters with an infected person even if there is no sexual contact, intravenous drug users, and people with multiple sexual partners (particularly men who have relations with men), people on hemodialysis, and anyone who needs blood products. You need a second shot one month after the first one, and a third shot six months later.

Hepatitis A This replaces the previously used gamma globulin shot. You need this immunization if you'll be traveling to certain areas abroad. The best plan is to get two shots six months apart, but you'll be protected enough after one shot to leave right away if necessary. Call to be sure your doctor has the medication on hand. You may need to get a prescription, buy the medication yourself, and bring it to the office so the nurse can give you the injection. The immunization is also recommended for food handlers, gay men, day care workers, health care workers, and people with chronic liver disease.

Polio Most Americans were immunized as children. If for some reason you weren't, discuss your options with your physician. There is some controversy over whether adults should get the vaccine at all. The inactivated virus (shot form) is safer and preferred.

Lyme Vaccine This is a newly available vaccine for people who live in high-risk areas where deer ticks carry lyme disease, a serious illness which can cause chronic arthritis.

Tuberculosis Skin Test (PPD) This is a test to see whether you've been exposed to the disease. It is NOT an immunization, but results should be recorded. Note: Some people test positive even though they don't have the disease. This means they are harboring the bacteria. Warning: They should consult with their doctor before taking steroids. A so-called new converter—a person who has previously tested negative and suddenly tests positive—will need to take medication as a preventive measure.

Travel to Foreign Countries If you're going to travel to foreign countries, call your local hospital to find out which shots you'll need based on your itinerary. You can also call the International Traveler's Hotline at the Centers for Disease Control (CDC), 888-232-3228, or visit www.cdc.gov or www.immunize.com.

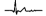

That was the easy part. Now we're going to move on to the screening and diagnostic exams and tests which can detect health problems early, yet which are not necessarily everybody's idea of a good time. But don't skip this section! What you're about to read is a pivotal part of my plan to help you save your own life.

TRIUMPHING OVER TEST ANXIETY

My friend Marlene tells me she knows she should go for a mammogram, but she keeps putting it off because she's afraid of finding out the worst. "It's like if I don't know, I don't have cancer," she says sheepishly. Marlene is a very together woman otherwise, but she's playing tricks on herself when it comes to her health. The truth, of course, is that finding out about a disease early gives you the best chance of beating it. What you don't know really *can* hurt you. Here are some tips on nudging yourself to get the tests you need:

1) Talk with your health buddy about your anxiety. Telling someone that you've been putting off scheduling a rectal exam or a blood test for prostate cancer is sure to bring home the fact that you're putting your health in jeopardy. Men traditionally have more of a problem than women do with talking about health concerns, so wives and women friends acting as health buddies may need to initiate a conversation—or leave this book open to page 75 or 107 on the coffee table!

2) Team up with your health buddy and make appointments for the same day, then go for your tests together. That will shore up your courage and keep you from "forgetting" or canceling. A mother and daughter I know decided to make a day of it when they were due for mammograms. They would dress up for the occasion and then have lunch together after the tests. One year, the daughter's X-rays showed suspicious changes. She was diagnosed with breast cancer at an early stage. Six years and one lumpectomy later, she is still very much alive—and very glad that she and her mother got each other to go for their mammograms without fail.

3) Reward yourself for going through with a test or exam. I have one friend who buys herself a little present—some

costume jewelry, a pretty scarf, a bottle of perfume—every year after she gets her pelvic/rectal exam and her Pap test. So far, she has had only good news. But she says she would treat herself even if the results showed something was wrong. She now realizes that she's gotten into a very good habit that could help her catch cancer and other problems early. That in itself is cause for celebration.

DOES IT RUN IN THE FAMILY?

Official guidelines such as those from the United States Preventive Services Task Force, the American Cancer Society, the Internal Medicine and Family Practice Organizations, the American Heart Association, and the American Diabetes Association may not be precise enough for you to use as your own yardstick. For one thing, those agencies have yet to reach a consensus and the jury is still out when it comes to when and how often some tests should be performed. More important, your family history is a potent predictor of your predisposition to certain diseases. You may need to have tests earlier or more often than the general population. So while I'm going to give some recommended ages and frequencies as I detail each test and procedure, I want you to take the time to write down your family health history. You'll get an individualized picture of your genetic risk factors. When you show this to your doctor, she will be able to help you decide whether to have screening tests and exams sooner than you might have if you had been going by the general recommendations.

Who to profile: Your mother, father, brothers, sisters, maternal grandmother, maternal grandfather, paternal grandmother, and paternal grandfather. You can also profile aunts, uncles, cousins, and great-grandparents if their health history contributes to your risk factors.

72

Step 4: Learning Which Immunizations, Exams, and Tests You Need

What to write about each family member: Give current age if living. If deceased, give age of death (approximate is fine if you don't know for sure) and cause of death if you know it. Then list for each family member any significant conditions and the age of onset as nearly as you can recall. The reason is that you should be screened for certain diseases when you are a few years younger than your relative was when he or she was diagnosed. Examples of what to list: diabetes, heart disease, liver or pancreas problems, kidney stones, arthritis, Alzheimer's, depression, and alcoholism. Also list lifestyle factors such as smoking, obesity, and lack of exercise.

THE WAY YOU LIVE

Along with your family history, you may have some risk factors associated with your lifestyle which will help your doctor individualize your prevention schedule. Be sure to take into consideration obesity or being overweight, lack of regular exercise, and excessive alcohol use. (Moderate alcohol use may actually be beneficial.) Smoking, of course, is another risk. Your doctor will want to know your "pack years." Multiply the number of packs a day (ppd) you smoke, or smoked, by the number of years. If you smoked two packs a day from the age of twenty to the age of forty, you racked up forty pack years. Your occupational history may be significant as well. And your age and gender are contributing factors.

As I said, your prevention schedule will be unique. However, I'm going to list and explain the routine exams and screening tests you should have at some point, and also discuss the diagnostic tests your doctor may order if your symptoms or test results suggest a problem.

ROUTINE PHYSICAL EXAMS YOU NEED
General Physical

Purpose

Your doctor can tell a great deal about your health by talking to you, looking at you, and examining areas of your body. She will also check your blood pressure, height, and weight. She'll probably order blood work and do a urinalysis.

Getting Ready for the Test

You don't need to do anything special before your exam. However, if you have collected your health records, bring them with you. You will be asked to give a urine sample, so don't urinate right before you're about to see the doctor.

What to Expect

Some doctors will talk with you before the physical exam. Others will do the exam first and then talk with you. Whenever the talking happens, this is what it will entail: The doctor will do a review of systems (ROS), which is an orderly way of taking your medical history and eliciting information from you about how you feel and about what prompted the visit. The review also includes your doctor's own subjective observations about you, such as whether you appear younger or older than your chronological age, whether you look sallow or seem to be fatigued. She has been trained to do this part of the exam from head to toe so she won't forget or miss anything.

The physical exam also goes from head to toe, and your doctor has been trained to work from the right side of the examining table. Before the physical exam, you'll be asked to undress, put on a gown, give a urine sample, and go sit on the table. The nurse will probably come in to weigh you, test your urine sample with a chemical strip (see page 88), draw blood from your arm (see page 79), and take your vital signs, which include blood pressure (see page 78), your pulse, and an EKG (see page 95). Then the doctor will check the following: 1) your skin, to see if there are moles, rashes, or signs of melanoma, 2) your lymph nodes to detect swelling, 3) the HEENT series, which includes your head, eyes, ears, nose, and throat, 4) the "Cor," which is Latin for heart, 5) your lungs, 6) your abdomen, 7) your extremities, 8) your genitourinary tract (GU, men only; GYN, women only), 9) your rectum, 10) and your neurologic functions including mental status via a recall test and your reflexes. During these tests, your doctor will use her gloved hands as well as standard tools such as a lighted instrument to check your eyes and ears, a tongue depressor to see your throat, a stethoscope to listen to your heart, and a rubber hammer to test your reflexes.

After the exam, the doctor will come to some conclusions about what your symptoms, if any, may mean. She will then talk with you about your treatment options and about lifestyle changes which could help you.

When and How Often

If you're generally healthy, have a complete head-to-toe exam every three to five years, and once a year after age sixty-five. Some parts of the complete physical should be done more often, as follows:

Rectal

Purpose

For both men and women, this is a preliminary test for

colon cancer. For men, it is also a way to palpate the prostate, and for women it is a way to palpate the pelvic organs.

Getting Ready for the Test

You don't need to do anything special before your exam.

What to Expect

A man will be asked to lie on his left side on the examining table, as will a woman if the exam is not part of a pelvic. A woman also having a pelvic will be asked to lie on her back. Using lubricating gel, the doctor will insert a gloved finger into your rectum. Men may sense the need to urinate. Breathe deeply and relax. It will be over in a matter of seconds.

When and How Often

Every year or so after age forty and yearly after age fifty.

Pelvic (For Women Only)

Purpose

Your doctor will check for enlargement of the uterus and ovaries and abnormalities of the cervix and vagina. He can also take a smear to check for two sexually transmitted diseases, chlamydia and gonorrhea.

Getting Ready for the Test

Empty your bladder right before the exam.

What to Expect

While you're lying on your back on the examining table with your feet in the stirrups, the doctor will insert a device called a speculum into your vagina. This allows her to see the walls of the vagina and the opening of the cervix and take a sample for the Pap smear. She can't use a lubricant until after the cell sample has been taken. A metal speculum will probably feel cold. The disposable plastic type won't, but some doctors feel it doesn't function as well. After the cell sample has been taken, your doctor will insert a lubricated gloved finger and use the other hand on your abdomen. This won't hurt at all.

When and How Often

Have this exam once a year from the time you're sexually active.

Breast

Purpose

Your doctor will check your breasts for lumps and abnormalities that could signal cancer.

Getting Ready for the Test

You don't need to do anything special before your exam. The best time to be checked is the week after your period starts, when your breasts are less glandular and lumpy.

What to Expect

While you're lying on your back and then sitting on the examining table, the doctor will gently press on your breasts.

When and How Often

From the age of eighteen on, you need a professional exam ideally once a year. You also should examine your own breasts once a month during the week after you get your period. After menopause, you can do your exam any time of the month. If you pick a certain day such as the first of the month and note that on your calendar, you'll be less likely to forget. Also, any man who notices a lump should see his physician.

ROUTINE SCREENING TESTS YOU NEED
Blood Pressure

Purpose

Your blood pressure is taken to find out whether you have hypertension, also known as high blood pressure. This condition is a big risk factor for heart disease, stroke, and kidney failure.

Getting Ready for the Test

Often a patient who gets a high reading will tell me that he's just stressed out, both by being in a doctor's office and by facing the possibility of bad news. If the patient who says something like that is overweight, over fifty, sedentary, and a smoker, I have to be skeptical. But some people's blood pressure really might shoot up because of nerves and therefore give a false reading. So breathe deeply and try to stay calm. If you know how to meditate, do so. Also, your blood pressure will rise during vigorous exercise, so don't dash into the doctor's office right after a workout at the gym.

What to Expect

A cuff will be wrapped fairly snugly around your upper arm and then inflated via a squeezable bulb. The process may be repeated a couple of times and sometimes on both arms.

When and How Often

From the age of five on, everyone should have his or her

blood pressure checked once every two or three years. If yours is high, your doctor will recommend more frequent checks. You can test your own pressure fairly reliably at home with devices available at pharmacies and through mail order health catalogues. This should not be a substitute for a professional exam, however.

Understanding Your Test Results

Systolic pressure comes first and diastolic comes second. Systolic is always the higher number of the two. Both are measured in millimeters of mercury, in the same way that a thermometer uses mercury. The new digital devices don't use mercury, but the traditional mercury-based numbers are used anyway.

Systolic means the pressure in the arteries when the heart is beating. The norm is less than 140, or less than 160 if you're over sixty-five. The lower the number, the better. Diastolic means the pressure in the artery when the heart is at rest between beats. The norm is 60–85, and again, the lower the better.

Blood Work

Purpose

Your blood contains a great deal of information about your health. When your doctor orders the lab to run a complete series of tests, you can find out about the status of your liver, your thyroid, your blood sugar, your cholesterol, and much more. The tests can also be a clue to infections, internal bleeding, and some forms of cancer such as leukemia.

Getting Ready for the Test

Usually, you don't have to prepare for a blood test, but your doctor may ask you to skip breakfast if she's looking for something specific such as diabetes or high cholesterol. Your blood sugar and blood fats remain high for a couple of hours after you eat.

What to Expect

The technician will wrap a tourniquet around your upper arm and draw blood with a syringe from a vein inside your elbow. She will probably draw two samples. After she's finished and has put a Band-Aid on the spot where the syringe went in, raise your arm and press firmly on that spot for at least thirty seconds with your other hand. This will prevent you from ending up with a nasty-looking bruise.

The blood the technician draws goes directly into color-coded tubes with special preservatives. Blood drawn into a lavender-topped tube is for your complete blood count (CBC). Blood drawn into a red-topped tube is used to check your blood chemistry.

When and How Often

The general recommendation is to have at least your cholesterol checked every five years after the age of twenty. However, a complete blood "panel" doesn't cost much more and it may reveal unexpected abnormalities. Also, if you have family or lifestyle risk factors for any given condition, you should be tested accordingly.

Understanding Your Test Results

Many doctors will mail you a form with such categories as sugar, liver function, and cholesterol, and columns with check marks indicating whether the test results are normal or abnormal. That's not good enough. Remember Jeremy back in Step 3, the teenager whose sugar was checked as being "normal" even though it was far below normal? His mother found that out when she asked for and studied a copy of the original test results from the laboratory. This is an example of why it's vital for you to hold your test results in your own hands. Even more to the point, some doctors don't even send out the dumbed-down forms. They let you believe that no news is good news and that you'll hear from them only if there's a problem. The trouble is that no news very often is simply no news. Your results may have been lost or accidentally placed in someone else's file, or your doctor may have given the results only a quick glance and missed something.

Understanding your own results isn't all that difficult. People always tell me that looking at their numbers is, to use an overworked but perfect word, "empowering." If your cholesterol breakdown is bad news, you can start researching possible causes and ways to manage the problem. Then later if your numbers improve, you'll feel as though you just got an A on your report card. That will motivate you to stay with the program, whereas reading the word "normal" would have been the emotional equivalent of getting a pass grade in a pass/fail system.

The results of your blood tests will be printed in columns headed "In Range" and "Out of Range." Next to that is a column called the "Reference Range," which means the numbers that are normal. The reference range can vary from lab to lab, so always compare your current results with the reference range on your current report only. There are a few absolutes such as cholesterol, CBC, and glucose, but in general there is no standardized reference range. Note: The blood in the red-topped tube is spun in a centrifuge to separate the clotted cells from the liquid or serum. The laboratory uses only your serum for blood chemistry tests such as sugar and liver function. It can also check for syphilis and

HIV, so request these results if you have reason to be concerned. If the blood is collected or spun improperly, the results can be wildly inaccurate across the board. You'll need to go back and give another sample to get a true reading.

Here are the main categories you'll see on your copy of the test results:

Complete Blood Count (CBC)

This is the most common blood test. Your doctor may order it as part of a complete physical examination. He'll also order it before you have surgery and if you have unexplained symptoms. The CBC measures the number, size, and shape of the different types of cells in your blood. The clinically important ones are as follows:

Hemoglobin measures whether your red blood cells have enough of the protein which carries oxygen. If your count is low, you have anemia. The normal range for women is 12–14 grams and for men it's 14–16.

Hematocrit shows the ratio of red blood cells to your total blood volume. It's reported as a percentage. If yours is low, you have anemia. The norm for women is 36 percent and for men it's 42 percent. Doctors figure it by tripling the hemoglobin in the same way you would double a 7.5 percent tax on your restaurant bill to arrive quickly at a 15 percent tip.

Mean Corpuscular Volume (MCV) gives the size and shape of your red blood cells. If you have anemia, the results give your doctor a clue to the type. For example, small cells indicate iron deficiency and some hereditary anemias such as sickle cell and thalassemia. Large cells show nutritional deficiencies such as low B_{12} or folate.

White Blood Cell Count (WBC) is exactly what it says. Because white blood cells increase as part of your immune response, a high count could signal that your body is fighting an infection. Other causes of an elevated WBC are chronic inflammation, stress, recent vigorous exercise, and certain medications including steroids.

Differential White Blood Cell Count shows whether your percentage of each of the six types of white blood cells is within the normal range. If your WBC is abnormal, the differential can help your doctor zero in on the cause. For example, a high level of the type of white blood cell called segmented neutrophils usually points to a bacterial infection rather than a viral infection.

Platelet Count shows whether you have enough of the cells which help your blood clot properly. (This has nothing to do with hemophilia, a hereditary disorder in which coagulating proteins are deficient.) Various factors such as stress, alcohol abuse, and iron deficiency can affect your platelet count. If it's low, you'll bruise and bleed too easily. Knowing your platelet count before undergoing surgery is obviously important.

Erythrocyte Sedimentation Rate (ESR or SED Rate) measures how fast your red blood cells settle to the bottom of a tube during a one-hour period. Severe anemia, infection, chronic inflammation disorders, and some cancers can cause the cells to settle faster than normal and give an elevated result. Note: Women's cells naturally settle faster than men's do.

Blood Chemistry

A single sample of your blood serum can be used to run a series of tests quickly and inexpensively. However, many insurance plans won't reimburse you unless your doctor justifies ordering all the chemistry tests by listing a numerical code for your diagnosis or medical condition. The following explains the most commonly requested tests:

Glucose (Blood Sugar) can indicate diabetes if your level is high or hypoglycemia if it's low.

Blood Urea Nitrogen (BUN) and Creatinine are tests of your kidney function. Even a minor elevation of creatinine, the waste product of your muscles, can signal early kidney problems. The smaller your muscle mass, the lower your creatinine should be within the normal range. Even when it stays in the normal range, however, it could signal the beginning of kidney disease if it doubles from your previous results.

Sodium, Potassium, and Chloride are blood salts, or electrolytes. These tests are especially important if you are on diuretics ("water pills") for hypertension, since you can lose potassium.

Uric Acid is a waste product of all cells. An elevated level may mean kidney disease or gout, which is a hereditary form of arthritis exacerbated by certain diets and alcohol. If you take diuretics, your count may be high. If you have no symptoms of gout, kidney disease, or kidney stones, your doctor may not suggest any further treatment.

Albumin is a blood protein produced by your liver. A low albumin count can be a sign of liver or kidney disease or malnutrition.

Globulin is a blood protein produced by your immune system. A high count can point to chronic inflammation, infection, or blood disorders such as multiple myeloma.

Calcium is a component of your blood which helps all the cells in your body function normally. Unless you consume enough calcium in your diet or through supplements, your body will take calcium from your bones in order to keep the blood level in the normal range. This puts you at risk for osteoporosis, or brittle bones that break easily. Remember, though, that your blood calcium level has nothing to do with how much calcium is in your bones. A high count doesn't have anything to do with how dense your bones are, and in fact it can point to a disorder called hyperparathyroidism which predisposes you to kidney stones as well as osteoporosis.

Serum Glutamine Pyruvic Transaminase (SGPT) and Serum Glutamate-Oxaloacetate Transaminase (SGOT) SGOT and SGPT are enzymes (proteins) produced primarily by the liver. SGOT is also produced by red blood cells. Both SGOT and SGPT can be abnormally high if you have liver disease. Mild increases in these two enzymes can alert your doctor to look for asymptomatic liver conditions including inflammation caused by certain medications, obesity, or alcoholism. Another possibility is hemochromatosis, a treatable hereditary condition in which you store too much iron.

Lactate Dehydrogenase (LDH) is an enzyme produced by many cells of the body. If this test is extremely high, your doctor will want to do additional tests, depending on your specific complaints, to rule out malignancies.

Bilirubin is the chemical in bile that gives it the yellow color. When the bile passage from the liver to the intestine is blocked, your bilirubin level will be high. Possible causes are gallstones and liver disease. A symptom is jaundice, a yellowing of the skin and the whites of the eyes. Some people have a harmless hereditary condition, Gilbert's syndrome, in which the bilirubin is always a little high. A clue that you have this condition is a high bilirubin level every time your blood is tested. This is another example of why saving all your results and carrying a list of your medical conditions in your wallet is important. If you end up in an emergency room with abdominal pain, doctors won't waste time looking for liver problems simply because your bilirubin is a little high. They'll check your liver, but they'll move right on to looking for other causes of your pain as well.

Gamma Glutamyl Transpeptidase (Gamma-GGT) is an enzyme produced by the liver. Obesity and excessive alcohol use are the most common reasons it can be mildly increased. It will also be elevated when there is blockage of bile, and with liver disease.

Blood Fats

Also called lipids, these are often listed together in a separate "panel" on your blood chemistry report. Sometimes only the total cholesterol and perhaps the triglyceride level will be listed if your doctor didn't specifically request results for the lipid panel. However, you need all your numbers (your "breakdown") in order to make the best evaluation of your risk for heart disease.

Total Cholesterol is the sum of your LDL, HDL, and triglycerides (see below). High total cholesterol levels are linked to heart disease. The lower your total cholesterol the better. Under 200 is desirable.

High Density Lipoprotein (HDL) is your "good cholesterol." Remember that "high density should be high." The more of this type, the better. Ideally, your HDL cholesterol should be at least 30 percent of your total amount. Women naturally have higher levels than men, although they have less of an advantage after menopause. Heredity, a sedentary lifestyle, and smoking can lower the level somewhat. A healthy diet won't change your HDL very much, but it will lower your total cholesterol.

Low Density Lipoprotein (LDL) is your "bad cholesterol."

Remember, "low density should be low." A high LDL puts you at risk for heart disease. An LDL of 130 or less is considered normal, but if you already have heart disease your doctor will suggest diet and often medication to get your LDL cholesterol below 100. Here are the recommended goals:

*Under 160 if you have no other risk factors for heart disease.

*Under 130 if two or more of the following apply to you: 1) smoking, 2) overweight, 3) inactivity, 4) diabetes, 5) a systolic blood pressure over 140, 6) a diastolic blood pressure over 90, 7) an HDL under 35, 8) a close female relative who had heart disease before age fifty-five, 9) a close male relative who had heart disease before age forty-five, 10) you are a male over forty-five, 11) you are a female over fifty-five, particularly if you're not taking estrogen.

*Under 100 if you have heart disease.

Triglycerides are the main form of fat in your blood. The level will be much higher after a meal. If your level is out of range, it should be rechecked after an overnight fast. Elevated levels increase your risk of heart disease, but not to the same degree as the cholesterol. High sugar diets and excessive alcohol consumption contribute to an elevated triglyceride level. Weight loss and cutting down on sugar and alcohol lower the level. Occasionally the level is so high that your doctor will suggest medication.

Thyroid Evaluation (Thyroid Function Tests) measures the level of two hormones produced by the thyroid gland: thyroxine 3 (T3) and thyroxine 4 (T4). They regulate your metabolism. The brain keeps your levels normal by sending the thyroid-stimulating hormone (TSH) to the thyroid gland if your T3 and T4 are low. If your thyroid is underactive or "slow," your T3 and T4 levels will be low and your TSH level will be high. If your thyroid is overactive or "too fast," your T3 and T4 will be high and your TSH will be low or unmeasurable. The TSH level is the single best indicator of the condition of your thyroid gland and the effects of thyroid medication.

Urinalysis

Purpose

A chemical analysis of your urine can reveal signs of a variety of disorders and can serve as corroboration if your blood work points toward similar problems. A microscopic examination of cells may offer clues to infections or cancer of the bladder or kidney.

Getting Ready for the Test

When the nurse asks you for a urine sample, wash the area around your urethra so that you can get a "clean catch." Begin by letting the first urine flow into the toilet to wash out the urethra. Then let the rest of the urine go into the cup the nurse will have given you. This way, your sample won't be contaminated.

What to Expect

The nurse may do a urinalysis immediately with a chemical strip. Also your doctor will either check the sample under a microscope or send it to a lab. If you have symptoms of an infection, your doctor may order a urine culture to check for growth of bacteria.

When and How Often

There are no specific recommendations. The test is usually done during a complete physical or when a patient has symptoms.

Understanding Your Test Results

Small amounts of blood in your urine may simply mean that you have just exercised vigorously or that you're menstruating, but your doctor will want to rule out the possibility of cancer. Albumin in your urine can signal early kidney disease. Glucose in your urine can be a sign of diabetes.

Stool Occult Blood or Fecal Occult Blood Tests (FOBT)

Purpose

This test is designed to find hidden (occult) blood in your stool. The blood can signal precancerous or cancerous polyps in the colon, or intestinal bleeding from such causes as a stomach ulcer, internal hemorrhoids, or severe colitis.

Getting Ready for the Test

Don't take aspirin or ibuprofen before the test because they can cause stomach bleeding. Don't eat horseradish, melons, or turnips because they can give you a false positive. Menstrual blood looks just like occult blood in the results, so wait until after your period. Conversely, high doses of vitamin C can *mask* occult blood, so stop taking it before the test.

What to Expect

Your doctor will give you a kit with three chemically impregnated stool cards. At home, you'll use a stick to smear a card with a stool sample three days in a row or three bowel movements in a row, whichever comes first. (The small amount of stool on the toilet paper is plenty for an adequate smear.) Cancers and polyps bleed intermittently, so one sample is not enough. Then you'll send the cards back to the doctor in the envelope that came with the kit. Note: If you have had rectal bleeding, even if it's probably just from hemorrhoids or fissures, there's no need to test for hidden blood. You need a sigmoidoscopy or a colonoscopy (see the following pages).

When and How Often

If you're over fifty, you should do this test every year. If you have a family history of polyps, colon cancer, or severe colitis, begin doing the test five years earlier than the age of onset of the disease for any family member.

Understanding Your Test Results

When your doctor puts a drop of a chemical onto the stool cards, hidden blood will turn the stool smears blue immediately. The cause may be precancerous polyps or internal bleeding, often from hemorrhoids (varicose veins of the anus), which is not a concern. In a small percentage of patients, the cause may be cancer. Your doctor will recommend further tests to make the diagnosis.

Sigmoidoscopy

Purpose

This is a screening procedure to detect polyps and colon cancer.

Getting Ready for the Test

I tell my patients to skip breakfast on the morning of the test and to give themselves a Fleet's enema (phosphate solution available without a prescription) or two before coming to the appointment. Your doctor may have different instructions, so be sure to ask what he recommends.

What to Expect

Your doctor may do this test himself, or he may refer you

to a gastrointestinal specialist. While you are lying on your left side, the doctor will insert a flexible tube about the size of your finger into your rectum. He will slowly pass the tube up at least 60 centimeters (29 inches), all the while pumping air to keep the passage open for visibility. The air can cause cramping, but you'll pass it as soon as the test is over. The test takes about ten to twenty minutes.

The flexible tube is called a sigmoidoscope. It is fiberoptic and lighted so the doctor can see polyps, tumors, or other abnormalities such as the pouches that indicate diverticulosis.

When and How Often

If you're over fifty, you should have this test every three to five years. If you have a family history of colon or rectal cancer, request the test when you are five years younger than your family member was at the time the disease was diagnosed. Also, if you have symptoms such as rectal bleeding, you should request this test no matter what your age or family history.

Understanding Your Test Results

A report of the sigmoidoscopy will be sent to your doctor if you went to a specialist. Otherwise, your doctor will sketch a diagram and write his own report. Ask for a copy and read it yourself. The report should include how far the scope was passed. If the tube was only passed 10 to 15 centimeters because of muscle spasm during the test or too much stool being present, the doctor didn't get a good look. You may need to have the test again. If the tube went in far enough, the doctor will either say that your colon looks normal, or he'll describe any abnormalities and recommend further testing if necessary such as a colonoscopy (see below).

Colonoscopy

Purpose

This is a diagnostic procedure to detect polyps, colon cancer, or any problems of the colon.

Getting Ready for the Test

Your doctor will refer you to a gastrointestinal specialist for this test, which is anything but fun. Still, it can save your life, so please don't avoid it! Here's the drill: Plan to take a day off work. The night before, you'll have to drink up to a gallon of a cherry-flavored laxative solution. It will taste best if you keep it cold. Drink a glass every fifteen minutes until you're finished. (Some doctors use a phosphate solution which is more concentrated, so you'll need to drink less.) You'll be running to the bathroom every ten to twenty minutes or so. This will, needless to say, clean out your colon. Don't eat or drink anything, except maybe little sips of water, after midnight. Skip breakfast.

If you have a heart valve condition or artificial joint, be sure to let the specialist know when you schedule the appointment. You may need intravenous antibiotics before the test, especially if a biopsy of the colon is likely. Also, your doctor will order routine pre-op blood work.

What to Expect

Just as in a sigmoidoscopy, a fiber-optic tube is inserted in your rectum. However, this one is long enough so that the doctor can see the entire length of your large colon. If a biopsy is to be performed, a loop will be inserted to snare a polyp or abnormal tissue. Because the scope and loop are passed so far up, you'll be given an intravenous sedative such as Versed and a painkiller such as Demerol. The former induces "retrograde amnesia" so that you won't remember having the test even though you'll be awake the whole time. The effects of the drugs will wear off fairly quickly. However, you will be groggy for a while and you must bring your health buddy along to drive you home.

When and How Often

This is a diagnostic procedure, not a routine screening test. You will have it when significant symptoms of the colon are present, or because of a family history of colon cancer, or when results of a stool fecal occult blood or sigmoidoscopy warrant further testing.

Understanding Your Test Results

The report from your colonoscopy may say that there were no polyps present. If there were polyps, and if a biopsy was done, you'll get a report from the lab (pathology). This will indicate the type of polyps you have. Those called "hyperplastic" are not premalignant and don't necessarily mean that you'll have any more polyps in the future. Those called "adenomatous" are precancerous and usually hereditary. If you have them, you're at risk for growing more polyps and developing colon cancer. You will be advised to be checked in one year, and then every three to five years after that.

Chest X-Ray

Purpose

Although the chest X-ray was originally devised to diagnose tuberculosis, it is now used to detect many conditions such as lung cancer, pneumonia, and heart enlargement. Common reasons your doctor may order a chest X-ray include preoperative screening, advanced age, and any unexplained symptoms such as chronic cough, chest pain, and shortness of breath.

Getting Ready for the Test

Take off all metal jewelry and your watch.

What to Expect

The technician will take front and side views, asking you to fully expand your lungs by taking a deep breath and holding it each time.

When and How Often

This is not a routine test. See "Purpose" above for symptoms and indications.

Understanding Your Test Results

Your doctor will get a copy of the radiologist's written report, but not the actual pictures. Comparing films from previous tests helps radiologists interpret current ones, so you may want to contact the X-ray department at the previous hospital and get your films. This is especially important if you move or if an abnormality is found.

Read your entire report, not just the conclusion. Sometimes the radiologist will see a shadow that does not look serious—such as one probably caused by your nipple. But it's your body, and "probably" isn't good enough. Ask your doctor if further X-rays or other tests are needed to rule out cancer.

The first part of your radiologist's report, called the "Comment Section," will describe in detail what he saw when he looked at your lungs, heart, mediastinum (where the major blood vessels and lymph nodes are located), and bones. There will be references to two views: posterior/anterior (PA), which means back and front; and lateral, which means side. Typical phrases you might see are "lungs well expanded," "presence of granulomas" (usually old scar tissue from previous infections), and "cardiovascular silhouette normal" or "cardiovascular silhouette enlarged." The radiologist will also note whether prior chest X-rays were available for comparison.

The second section, usually called the "impression," is the radiologist's opinion regarding what your X-rays show about your health. It is common for the radiologist to describe a normal chest X-ray as revealing "no active (disease) process."

Electrocardiogram (ECG or EKG)

Purpose

This test records your heart rhythm and detects heart damage and thickening of the heart muscle due to high blood pressure.

Getting Ready for the Test

You don't have to prepare for the test.

What to Expect

While you're lying on the examining table, the nurse will apply gel pads to areas on your arms, legs, and across your chest. Hair may need to be shaved first. Then electrode wires attached to a machine will be attached to the gel pads on your skin. The EKG machine measures the electrical activity of twelve different angles or views of your heart. You won't feel a thing. After the test, which takes only a minute or two, the nurse will take off the electrodes.

When and How Often

When indicated because of symptoms or health history, or prior to surgery.

Understanding Your Test Results

This is one instance in which you probably won't be able to interpret the test results yourself. You may have seen an EKG printout before. It looks like a graph with peaks and valleys. Your doctor will tell you if anything is unusual. Also note that today's sensitive computers often pick up the slightest variation from the norm, so you may see the word "abnormal" on your printout even if you're perfectly healthy. Note: Ask your doctor to reduce the size of your printout on a copy machine. Then carry it with you so anyone treating you would know what is normal for you.

Cardiac Stress Test

Purpose

This is an EKG that is taken while you are exercising on a treadmill. The purpose is to find out how your heart performs when you're exerting yourself. Even if the electrical activity of your heart and the blood flow to your heart are normal when it is at rest and beating slowly, if your arteries are blocked there may not be enough blood passing through when your heart rate increases. In that case, abnormal electrical activity will show up during the stress test.

Getting Ready for the Test

You'll be asked not to eat for at least three hours prior to the test. If you are on medications, you can take them on schedule unless your doctor advises you not to do so. Plan to wear comfortable shoes and clothing. If you're coming from the office, bring your gym bag and change into sweats and sneakers.

What to Expect

Cardiologists have the equipment for doing an exercise test. However, if you need the radioactive material thallium (see below), you'll need to go to the hospital as an outpatient. Plan on spending at least half a day away from work or other responsibilities. There are no showers available, so consider going home before you go back to the office if you tend to break a sweat easily.

Before you step up on the treadmill and start walking, the nurse will attach electrodes just as she would if this were a resting EKG. Also, if your resting EKG showed problems, your doctor may request that a harmless radioactive material such as thallium be injected intravenously right after the test. An X-ray will be taken at that time, and again four hours later. (Bring something to read in between.)

You will probably walk for ten to twenty minutes to get to your target heart rate, which is a number determined by such factors as your age, gender, height, and weight. The incline of the treadmill will become gradually steeper during the test, making the exercise more of a challenge. If you experience chest pain, leg pain, fatigue, or shortness of breath during the test and/or have changes in your electrical activity, the technician will stop the test before you get to your target rate because continuing could be risky.

When and How Often

To diagnose or monitor a heart problem.

Understanding Your Test Results

You need to get at least 85 percent of your target heart

rate in order to have a reliable reading. The faster your heart rate, the more likely it is that any blockage will show up on the EKG. If your rate only went up to 70 percent or 80 percent of your predicted rate because you got winded and had to stop, your heart wasn't worked enough. Your doctor may do another test using medication to speed up your heart. Note: For some reason, women more often than men have positive (abnormal) stress test results, yet when their arteries are checked with dye or catheters, they turn out to be free of blockage.

Your blood pressure will go up during the exercise test, which is normal. If it doesn't, that may point to a problem. The peak exercise heart rate and blood pressure are usually recorded. If your blood pressure goes down, this can signal a serious blockage or weakness of the heart and is worrisome. This test will also show what kind of condition you are in, referred to on your report as your "functional capacity." If your heart rate rose significantly before you walked very long and before the incline was very steep, you are not in very good shape.

If you had radioactive X-rays, a separate report from the radiology nuclear medicine department will be sent. The radioactive material may show areas of the heart that are damaged or not getting enough blood following the exercise. This will help determine whether any electrical changes on your EKG are significant.

Ultrasonography (Ultrasound Scanning or Sonogram)
Purpose

Ultrasound tests are painless ways to detect abnormalities in a number of areas of the body, and to evaluate the health status of a fetus. In an echo ultrasound, waves bounce off dense tissues and create a shadow picture. For example, the echocardiogram displays a picture of the heart. The echo test given to pregnant women creates a picture of the unborn baby.

Doppler ultrasound tests use a microphone so that you and the clinician can hear the distinctive sound of blood flowing through an abnormal heart valve, or hear the sound of a fetal heartbeat.

Ultrasound is commonly used to detect heart and blood vessel problems such as mitral valve prolapse, thickening of the heart muscle, irritation of the lining of the heart, heart murmurs, enlarged hearts, blocked arteries and aneurysms (ballooned segments of blood vessels which can rupture), and phlebitis (blood clots). Ultrasound is also useful in detecting problems in the abdomen (gallbladder, liver, pancreas, and kidney), the pelvic area (vagina, ovary, and uterus), and the rectum (prostate).

Getting Ready for the Test

Before an abdominal sonogram, don't eat, drink, or smoke for six hours prior to the exam. Note: The vaginal probe ultrasound has by and large taken the place of an earlier type of sonogram for the pelvic area which required drinking a gallon or more of liquid first.

What to Expect

A transducer, a device which produces sound waves of a frequency too high for humans to hear, is attached to a video monitor. Abdominal and breast scans are done by placing the transducer on the area to be tested. Pelvic scans are done either by placing the transducer on the abdomen or by inserting the transducer into the vagina. For a prostate scan, the transducer is inserted into the rectum. The sound waves penetrate painlessly and are converted into electrical impulses which create the sound or picture your doctor uses to help make a diagnosis. Incidentally, the technician is not allowed to comment on what she sees during the test, so don't get nervous just because she doesn't give you a thumbs-up on the spot.

When and How Often

Because ultrasound is not a screening test but a diagnostic test, your doctor will order one when it seems warranted because of symptoms, results of other tests, and your health history.

Understanding Your Test Results

Your radiologist or specialist will write a report about your ultrasound and send it to your doctor. Ask your doctor for a copy. The report will generally be easy to read.

Dual X-Ray Absorptiometry Scan (DEXA or DXA Scan)

Purpose

This is an X-ray which measures your bone density. Loss of density is a sign of osteopenia or osteoporosis.

Getting Ready for the Test

You can remain fully clothed, but you need to remove your belt.

What to Expect

While you are lying on a table with a support under your knees, the technician will take pictures of your spine and hip. You don't have to wear a protective shield and nothing will touch you. The amount of radiation is minimal.

Step 4: Learning Which Immunizations, Exams, and Tests You Need

When and How Often

All women over sixty-five and all postmenopausal women not taking hormone therapy should have the test at least once. Women, particularly postmenopausal women, are prone to osteoporosis (thin bones). However, men on steroids or other bone-robbing medications are also susceptible. Both men and women with a history of kidney stones are at risk. Women who have risk factors such as a family history should have the test before age sixty-five. When osteoporosis is caught early, corrective measures can keep it from getting worse.

Understanding Your Test Results

You'll see numbers comparing your bone density to that of a typical young person at peak bone mass, about age thirty-five. This is your T-score, the most important score to check. If your T-score results are between -1 and -2.5 points, you have the beginnings of bone loss, called osteopenia. If your T-score is -2.5 or more, you have osteoporosis. The lower the score, the greater the risk of fractures.

There will also be a column with the numbers for a normal population in your age and ethnic group. This is your Z-score. It's not nearly as significant as the T-score. You'll also see the percentage of bone you have lost—say 20 percent or 30 percent. This is often the only piece of information doctors give their patients, but it is not a particularly helpful way to describe the results and can't be used to assess your risk of fracture. Get the report and look at your T-score yourself. (There is no special reason these are called T- and Z-scores.)

Computed Tomography (CAT or CT) Scan

Purpose

A CAT scan is a type of X-ray developed during the 1970s which takes many more "slices" or views than a conventional picture. You will be exposed to more radiation than with a plain X-ray, but the extensive and detailed films which result can shed light on problems in many areas of the body and help your doctor make a diagnosis. Abdominal CAT scans have decreased the need for exploratory surgery because your doctor gets a good look inside of you without "opening you up."

There is a new test on the horizon called the "Ultra Fast CT of the heart." It shows calcium deposits in the coronary arteries, which may be an early sign of heart disease.

Getting Ready for the Test

If you're going to have a CAT scan of your abdomen, don't eat or drink anything for four to six hours prior to the examination. You'll be asked to drink up to a gallon of a flavored barium preparation while you're in the waiting room. The barium will show up on the X-ray as a distinct shadow, helping the radiologist distinguish between your bowel and other organs.

If you are allergic to iodine or X-ray dye, be sure to tell your doctor. During the procedure, a "contrast dye" may be injected intravenously to allow the doctor to see the blood vessels better. If this will be true in your case, your doctor can prescribe a combination of a steroid, a histamine blocker, and an antihistamine to prevent an adverse reaction to the dye. (Don't forget to note your iodine or contrast dye allergy on the list you carry in your wallet. See page 37).

Step 4: Learning Which Immunizations, Exams, and Tests You Need

What to Expect

You will be placed in a tube, but it is not entirely enclosed.

When and How Often

Only when indicated by symptoms and previous test results.

Understanding Your Test Results

The radiologist will send a typed report which is pretty much in plain English to your doctor. Ask for it. Check your reference books and medical dictionary (see Step 3) if you find terms you don't understand.

Magnetic Resonance Imaging (MRI) Scan

Purpose

An MRI scan is a type of X-ray that uses magnetic fields instead of radiation. Like a CAT scan, the MRI can "look" inside your body, but the images of soft tissues are often sharper. An MRI is often the preferred test when your doctor is looking for torn ligaments or torn cartilage, stress fractures, or internal tissue damage in the breast or brain.

Getting Ready for the Test

Tell your doctor if you have any metal implants such as staples or clips from previous surgery, or titanium in a prosthetic hip joint. Also, if you have gunshot pellets that were never removed, mention that. The metal could dislodge when it is pulled by the magnetic field, or interfere with the pictures because the X-ray can't penetrate metal.

Many people benefit from taking a sedative before an MRI.

What to Expect

You will lie down on something similar to an examining table. This table will then be moved into an enclosed cylinder. You must hold still for as long as twenty or thirty minutes. Now you know why you might want a sedative! In fact, if you're really claustrophobic, you may need to go to a facility that has open scanners.

When and How Often

When warranted by symptoms.

Understanding Your Test Results

The results are typed and easy to understand.

Bone Scan

Purpose

This test is not the same as the DEXA scan for bone density we discussed on page 100. A bone scan is a nuclear medicine test which can diagnose chronic osteomyelitis (infection in the bone), stress fractures, and bone cancer.

Getting Ready for the Test

Plan to take at least half a day if not a full day off work.

What to Expect

The doctor will inject a radioactive material intravenously, usually in your arm. You will then wait two or three hours while the material is taken up by your bones. You will not feel anything. Then you will go into a special room, get undressed, put on a gown, and lie on a table. The technician will use a scanner which counts radioactive material and prints a picture. The camera will not touch you.

When and How Often

When warranted by symptoms.

Understanding Your Test Results

The results are a picture of your skeleton with problems shown by the radioactive material as darker areas. Arthritis (inflammation of the joints) can give you a false positive, but the radiologist usually can tell the difference. There will be a written report.

Dental

Purpose

To check teeth for decay and plaque buildup; to probe gums for inflammation (gingivitis), excess mobility of teeth; to examine mouth for signs of cancer, diabetes, vitamin deficiencies, irregularities in bite, saliva, facial structure, and thermomandibular joint (TMJ).

Getting Ready for the Test

There is no special preparation for the checkup, but you should be practicing good oral hygiene all the time, including regular brushing and flossing.

What to Expect

The hygienist will clean, floss, and polish your teeth. The dentist will check your teeth, gums, and mouth and palpate your lymph nodes.

When and How Often

Every six months, or more often if you have problems such as excessive plaque or inflamed gums.

Understanding Your Test Results

They are not in plain English and you probably won't understand them. You can ask your dentist to translate if you have a particular concern.

Vision

Purpose

To check your vision and your eye muscles, and to screen for eye disease such as glaucoma, cataracts, macular degeneration, and diabetic retinopathy. Many eye diseases are asymptomatic.

Getting Ready for the Tests

Contact lens wearers will be asked to take out lenses about twenty minutes before the exam.

What to Expect

For some tests, drops are put in your eyes to dilate the pupils. A glaucoma test involves a puff of air into your eye to check for pressure. The rest of the exam involves resting your chin on a curved surface and looking through special lenses while you read eye charts.

When and How Often

Every two or three years up to age forty, and every one or two years from forty to sixty. After age sixty, annually. An optometrist does not have a medical degree, but is qualified to do your exam and dispense glasses or contact lenses. In the event that you need medication or surgery, your optometrist will refer you to an ophthalmologist.

Also, see an eye care specialist immediately if you experience loss or dimness of vision, eye pain, excessive discharge from the eye, double vision, or redness or swelling of the eyelid.

Understanding Your Test Results

These are largely abbreviations. Ask your doctor to explain anything you don't understand.

Prostate Specific Antigen (PSA) Test (For Men Only)

Purpose

Your doctor can order a blood test to measure the level of the protein produced by your prostate, the gland which secretes most of the fluid that makes up your semen. This test may detect early prostate cancer.

Getting Ready for the Test

There is no preparation needed.

What to Expect

This is ordered as part of the blood work in the red-topped tube. (See page 79.)

When and How Often

There are no definitive guidelines. You and your doctor can make a decision based on your risk factors such as heredity, race, your current age, and whether or not your prostate has begun the typical enlargement process that comes with aging.

Understanding Your Test Results

As the prostate enlarges, your PSA level may increase. Any number above 4 is considered abnormal and may mean further tests such as ultrasound or a biopsy are necessary. Also, even if the number falls in the normal range

107

but has doubled since your last test, that could be significant.

Pap Test (For Women Only)

Purpose

Named after George Papanicolaou, the doctor who developed it in the 1930s and 1940s, this test can detect infection and precancerous or cancerous lesions of the cervix, which is the neck of the womb that opens into the vagina.

Getting Ready for the Test

Avoid sexual intercourse or douching for up to forty-eight hours before the exam to prevent contamination from semen or the douche solution. Also, schedule your exam between periods. Menstrual blood can contaminate the cell sample.

What to Expect

During a pelvic exam (see page 76), your gynecologist will insert a wooden spatula and then a small brush into your vagina to collect cells off your cervix. You might feel a little cramp. The whole thing takes only a few seconds.

When and How Often

You should have a Pap smear every 1 to 3 years from the time you become sexually active. There is good evidence that cervical cancer may be caused by the human papillomavirus (HPV) and is therefore a sexually transmitted disease. If you ever have precancerous or cancerous lesions, you'll need to have a colposcopy (see page 109) and then Pap smears more frequently after that. Your doctor will tell you how often to schedule the test.

Understanding Your Test Results

After looking at your cells under a microscope, a clinician will type a report. The first section will be "Sample Adequacy." If not enough of the deep endocervical cells were collected, or if the sample was contaminated with blood or semen, the clinician can't do a proper reading. If you see the phrase "sample inadequate," you'll know you need to go back for another test.

The rest of your report will be a description of what the clinician saw, using the Bethesda System, which groups findings into six categories as follows: 1) normal, 2) infections, 3) reactive or reparative changes (probably not serious), 4) squamous cell abnormalities, which may or may not indicate precancerous lesions or cancer, 5) glandular cell abnormalities, which may or may not indicate cancer, and 6) cancer.

If your report shows significant abnormalities, your doctor will talk to you about your options. She'll probably suggest a colposcopy, which is a way of looking at your cervix through a magnifying lens. You may also need a biopsy. Note: It is possible to get false results from a Pap smear, but the test is accurate over 90 percent of the time.

Some laboratories now do a preliminary analysis of cervical cells with Pap Net, a computerized system for identifying abnormalities. If a possible problem is detected, a human clinician steps in and evaluates the slide. The Pap Net is expensive, and critics argue that the computer finds every little insignificant abnormality and causes patients to worry needlessly. On the other hand, proponents point out that relying solely on a technician who looks at hundreds of slides a day means that an occasional significant abnormal area may be missed. Even so, what is missed one year will in all probability be picked up the following year.

Precancerous changes take up to ten years to become malignant, so there's time to catch them while they're still treatable. The bottom line is that insurance companies probably won't pay for the additional cost of the computer analysis, so it's up to you to decide whether you want to pay the difference, about $50, or stick with the old-fashioned method.

Endometrial Biopsy (For Women Only)

Purpose

This test can detect endometrial cancer as well as a benign postmenopausal condition in which the endometrium (lining of the uterus) is too thick.

Getting Ready for the Test

You'll be asked to skip breakfast and take two or three ibuprofen tablets before your appointment to minimize cramping.

What to Expect

In the doctor's office, while you're lying on your back on the examining table, your doctor will pass a thin plastic catheter through the cervix into the uterus and extract some material. The process takes about ten minutes. You may feel minor cramping.

When and How Often

Annually if you are taking unopposed estrogen, or when symptoms such as unexplained postmenopausal bleeding warrant the test.

Understanding Your Test Results

The report will be fairly straightforward. As always, look up terms you don't recognize.

Mammogram

Purpose

A mammogram is an X-ray which may detect breast cancer early, often before a lump can be felt.

Getting Ready for the Test

If possible, schedule the test the week after you get your period, and avoid caffeine, which may cause the appearance of lumpiness in your breasts. It's best to wear a two-piece outfit. Some facilities request that you avoid the use of talcum powder, deodorant, and perfume prior to the test.

What to Expect

You'll undress and put on a gown. When your turn comes, the clinician will show you into a room with a large X-ray machine which has a bottom plate where she'll place your breast and a top plate which will be lowered to secure your breast in place. First, the clinician may put stickers on your nipples so the radiologist won't mistake a nipple shadow for a lump.

Having your breast clamped inside the plates of the machine is certainly not comfortable and may be painful, but the X-ray takes only seconds. You'll be asked to hold your breath, and then it will be over. The clinician will take two or three views of each breast and might do another series a few minutes later after the radiologist has a look at the pictures. Don't panic. Usually the problem is just that not enough of your breast could be seen on the original films, or that your breasts were not spread out enough. Many patients ask me whether the test breaks the breast tissue and makes the breasts sag. It doesn't. However, let the technician know if you have silicone implants because they could be broken. She needs to clamp your breasts as gently as possible.

When and How Often

The general guideline is to have a test every year or two from forty to fifty, and annually after fifty. You and your doctor can devise a special schedule if you have a family history of breast cancer. Note: A man who notices a breast lump should have this test.

Understanding Your Test Results

The radiologist will write a two-part report: 1) what he saw, and 2) his "impression" of what those observations mean. Read the whole thing because he might mention subtle abnormalities in the first part but conclude that nothing is awry. It's your breast and your job to question whether abnormalities warrant further testing. Remember Susan Henley back in Step 2?

Common terms you might see on your mammogram include:

Dense fibroglandular tissue This is a normal finding for many menstruating women and occasionally for women on HRT (hormone replacement therapy).

Scattered calcifications Breast tissue commonly contains tiny spots of calcium in a random pattern. This has nothing to do with your bones or your calcium supplements. Your body deposits calcium as a reparative response, so the scattered pattern usually indicates nothing more than previous breast inflammation and/or infections, often from breastfeeding. This finding won't change from year to year. New calcifications, especially if they appear in clusters, will alert you and your doctor to the possibility of cancer and the need for a breast biopsy.

Clinical correlation is required Because the mammogram has only an 85 percent accuracy rate for detecting cancer, the radiologist wants your doctor to assess your family history and risk factors and to do a breast exam or a biopsy to decide whether further testing would be prudent. In the same vein, if you or your doctor feel a lump in your breast, a breast ultrasound or a biopsy should be done even if your mammogram was normal. Better safe than sorry.

YOUR HEALTH CALENDAR

Now that you know which preventive measures you need, you can start a reminder calendar by noting when you should have your inoculations. You can also slot in any tests and exams for which you can follow the standard guidelines. Then after you have talked with your doctor about your risk factors, you can fill in the blanks.

Computer programs which create calendars with built-in repeat functions are ideal for this purpose because you can set them to remind you even five or ten years hence that you need a routine physical or a tetanus shot. If you're using a print calendar or a day book system, jot notes on the December page such as "Due for physical in 2005" or "Due for tetanus shot in 2010." Then when you get your calendar for the next year, copy the notes onto the new December page. At the end of 2004 or 2009, write the reminder on the January page.

Your health calendar should also be used to keep track of your appointments and of when you need to refill prescriptions. If you combine your health calendar with your general calendar, make the health notations in a special color so they stand out. On a computerized calendar, you can insert a visual reminder from the clip art—a doctor figure in a white coat or an R_x. The point is to make sure you have a system for keeping track of the dates when you need to act in order to safeguard your health. Nobody else in this day and age is going to do that for you.

You now have the self-confidence, the paperwork, and the knowledge you need to get the best care possible. Step 5 will teach you how to put all of that to good use when you're face-to-face with your doctor...

Step 5 Helping Your Doctor Help You

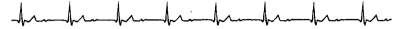

*"If you don't ask, your doctor might not tell.
If you don't tell, your doctor might not ask"*
— *Marie Savard, M.D.*

Bob and Laurie, dear friends of mine, volunteered to be a husband-and-wife tester team when I was developing my concepts for this book. I wanted to find out from the patient's perspective just what it would take to implement the step-by-step plan for saving your own life that I'm advocating. Bob was forty-nine and Laurie was forty-six at the time. They both basically felt fine. Neither one had been to a primary care physician for a physical or a referral in years, although Laurie had been going to her gynecologist for an annual exam and Pap smear.

Chances are you see yourself in that scenario, since it's surprisingly typical. People from all walks of life tend not to go to the doctor unless they get really ill. As Laurie put it, "I hate having a checkup. I've always got a good excuse to put it off. Like, I've packed on a few pounds and I want to wait until I slim down before I step on that scale in front of the nurse. Or I'm too busy to be sick right now, so I don't want to have any tests that might show I've got some problem I didn't know about." Bob agrees, although he adds that he knows this behavior amounts to health care roulette. "I take the car and the dog for checkups more often than I go to the doctor myself," he says. "As long as I feel pretty much okay, I can kid myself into thinking there's no need to spend time away from work. It seems like I always end up sitting for hours in the doctor's waiting room, and then comes the part where you get poked and prodded. And you have to listen to advice about quitting smoking or getting more exercise. Let's face it. Even a routine exam is not exactly a clambake. It's easy to find a reason not to go."

Clearly, Bob's and Laurie's avoidance tactics were not helping their doctors help them. I have a lot to share with you about how to interact and collaborate with your doctor to get the best health care possible. But you've got to make and keep appointments in the first place before my tips can do you any good. Long ago in a distant galaxy, doctors used to send postcards reminding you that you were due for a visit. Not anymore. That's why I hope you'll follow Bob's and Laurie's example. They conquered their doctorphobia and agreed to make appointments for checkups. But first, I asked them to take two months to start my system of preparing for optimum use of the precious little time patients usually get with their doctors. Here are the three facets of that system for you to put into practice as well.

YOUR HEALTH JOURNAL: HOW AND WHY TO KEEP ONE

Cicero, the Roman lawyer and orator, once said: "The competent physician, before he attempts to give medicine to his patient, makes himself acquainted not only with the disease which he wishes to cure, but also with the habits and constitution of the sick man." That's sage advice, but it's not always easy for physicians at the dawn of the twenty-first century to follow. The days when a family doctor with a fairly small practice had the time to chat up each patient and tease out information about the person's symptoms and lifestyle are long gone.

The solution? You have to take the initiative. By the time you get to an office visit, you need to have on paper and on the tip of your tongue every pertinent piece of information about your health and about the way you live. Keeping a health journal is the perfect way to accomplish this. You can track symptoms and have a running record of everything from weight gain or loss to vague complaints to side effects of medications. With that kind of a log at your disposal, you can help your doctor quickly spot patterns and zero in on possible problems. Remember, about 80 percent of what your doctor uses to make a diagnosis comes from what you tell her about yourself and your family history.

Interestingly, while Laurie liked the idea of keeping a health journal, she insisted at first that she was so fit that there wouldn't be anything to write down. As for Bob, he said he was too hassled to put yet another task on his to-do list. I suggested that they should both give the project a trial run for two weeks, and then tell me how they were doing. At the end of that time, I learned that in the great tradition of women being the secretaries for their families, Laurie had ended up writing both her own log and her husband's. "Hey, I send the Christmas cards, I remember all the birthdays and anniversaries, I know when the kids' soccer games are," Laurie said with only a touch of chagrin. "Why should this be any different?" Laurie is not the only one. Close to forty years after the rebirth of American feminism, statistics show that women still make most of the health care decisions for their children, spouses, parents, and themselves. In all fairness, though, plenty of men these days are seriously interested in health and vigor. *Men's Health*, a magazine launched in the 1990s, has been flying off the newsstands since its very first issue. Not only that, but men showed up in record numbers for screening tests after the news broke about Colin Powell's battle with prostate cancer, Darryl Strawberry's surgery for colon cancer, and Regis Philbin's treatment for heart disease.

In any case, Laurie was content to track Bob's health as well as her own and he was happy to have her do that. The results of the first two weeks of journaling surprised both of them. "My period was late and really heavy," says Laurie. "I see now that I wouldn't have paid much attention to that if I hadn't been keeping a diary. Maybe this is the beginning of menopause. Now I'm totally into having a written record." Laurie also noticed some low back pain that followed long periods of sitting at a desk, something she had never done until she took a job as a receptionist in a dentist's office a few months earlier. And she got a cold sore, a common occurrence for her, but it had never dawned on her to keep an ongoing account of just how common it was. "So I'm convinced this is a great idea," she concluded. "I see now that I'll be able to give the doctor a complete picture with dates and frequency of symptoms and stuff like that. Otherwise, if he had asked me how often I have cold sores, for example, I would have just said something like 'Now and then.'"

As for Bob, he let Laurie debrief him most nights at dinner. It turned out he was getting indigestion after lunch fairly often and she started asking him about stressful events that might have played into the problem. She made a note of that to help the doctor out. She and Bob also ended up having a long-overdue discussion about the problems he was having with a new boss who had been promoted over Bob's head, but that's another story. . .

Laurie stuck with the journal keeping and found that it

was quick and even kind of fun to do. I think you will, too. You don't have to write something every day. Just make dated entries of anything that might be significant such as the timing of your menstrual cycle, the pattern and type of headaches, changes in a mole, lack of your usual get-up-and-go, a tick bite even if it produces no symptoms at the time, or recurring bouts with "honeymoon cystitis." In addition, be your own detective by noting—as Laurie did with her long stretches of sitting at her desk and Bob's stressful events—anything that might be triggering symptoms. Was it that late-night bowl of jambalaya that brought on your heartburn? Does red wine precipitate a migraine attack? Does going to bed at the same time every evening help you conquer insomnia? Does a nightcap leave you with a feeling the next morning of not having slept well? Here is one area where you really don't need a medical degree to pinpoint cause and effect. Besides that, your doctor isn't there with you eating the Cajun food or drinking the red wine or downing the Scotch on the rocks. Only *you* know what you eat, drink, and do day in and day out. That's why *you* are in the prime position to figure out what's making you feel the way you feel. Not that you should come up with your own diagnosis. What seems like heartburn might be an ulcer or worse. But by giving your doctor every possible scrap of information, nicely organized in diary fashion, you're upping your chance of having her correctly nail whatever is wrong with you.

And certainly, if you have a chronic condition or a history of recurring episodes of any disorder, or if you're on medications, you should keep a meticulous health journal. Don't expect your doctor to remember every detail of your case. That may seem to go without saying, but I know from experience that it's not. I'll never forget Sally, twenty-seven, who had a history of a heart murmur from mitral valve prolapse, a benign congenital condition in which the heart valve is lax and blood washes back through it. Sally was told to take an antibiotic before every visit to the dentist. Dental work can trigger serious infections in people with Sally's condition. However, in spite of the possible dire consequences, there was one time when Sally didn't stop to refill her prescription for antibiotics before she rushed to the dentist with a painful cavity. She felt okay after the cavity was taken care of, and she put the incident out of her mind.

A month later, she came down with a low-grade fever and a skin rash. She went to the doctor but didn't mention that she hadn't taken the antibiotic. She assumed that if there were a connection between her current complaints and her mitral valve problem, her doctor would pick up on that. In the meantime, *he* assumed that anybody with a serious problem would follow through on doctor's orders. A full two weeks went by before the doctor finally quizzed her about recent dental visits and uncovered the real story. Diagnosis: a heart valve infection called subacute bacterial endocarditis. By that time, Sally was a very sick young woman. Who was to blame? Well, yes, the doctor should have gone over her chart and questioned her the first time she came in. But as I have said in another way before, what good is talking about that "should" after the fact? If Sally had kept a health journal, she would have been in a position to help her doctor get to the bottom of her problem immediately. As it was, Sally did survive but only after a long and entirely unnecessary illness.

A happier story involves fifty-two-year-old Maya, married to Carl, sixty-two. Maya started asking for copies of all of her medical records and those of her husband. She kept them on file, but she also made notes in their health journals about any test results that looked a little suspicious or varied from year to year. After one of Carl's visits, she noticed that his PSA, which predicts possible prostate cancer, had doubled since his previous test (see page 107). It was still not out of range and had been considered normal by Carl's doctor when he glanced at the current results without going back over earlier numbers. However, when Maya alerted the doctor, he asked Carl to come in for further testing. Result: Carl was diagnosed with prostate cancer at a very early stage and he was completely cured. This is an example of how a patient's own health journal became a call to action even after an overworked doctor had given only cursory attention to the patient's file.

LOOK UP YOUR SYMPTOMS BEFORE YOUR OFFICE VISIT

Once you have started keeping your health journal, do a little research on anything that seems out of the ordinary. That way you'll know whether or not you need immediate attention and you'll also know which concerns are worth mentioning to your doctor during a regular visit or, more important, writing on your wallet card for reference in an emergency situation. This can sometimes mean the difference between life and death.

Catherine, a sixty-four-year-old who slipped and broke her ankle, had a history of recurring phlebitis, a condition in which blood clots form in inflamed veins, and sometimes break loose and travel to the lung with fatal results. No one had ever told her that the tourniquet applied during orthopedic surgery would put her at high risk of developing the lethal blood clots—and she had never asked or researched her condition. She didn't mention the phlebitis to the surgeon, she had no written record of previous episodes, and she had not noted her condition on a list to be carried with her. A week after the operation, Catherine died. Yet if the surgeon had known about Catherine's phlebitis, he would have given her blood thinners. Should Catherine's doctor have told her about the link between a history of phlebitis and orthopedic surgery? Yes, in the best of all possible worlds. Did he do so? No. Yet again, though, pointing a finger at the doctor won't bring Catherine back. Wishing that doctors were aware of every little nuance about your case and that they will communicate all of that to you won't make it so. So take up the mantle yourself by keeping a health journal, researching your conditions, and making sure everyone who becomes involved in your care has your medical history including significant conditions and diseases, and a list of medications and allergies.

EXPLAIN WHY YOU'RE MAKING AN APPOINTMENT

When patients have acute problems or one of the red flag symptoms we talked about in Step 1, they either show up at the emergency room or call the doctor and say something like: "I have a blinding headache that came out of nowhere" or "There's a mole on my chest that keeps growing." However, when symptoms are less dramatic, patients tend not to mention them when they call for a visit. As a result, the office manager may not schedule enough time, and the doctor uses up precious minutes ferreting out patients' concerns.

You can avoid that scenario by reviewing your health journal, researching your symptoms, consulting your immunization and prevention flow chart, and looking at your family history before you call the doctor's office. That way, you'll be ready to explain exactly why you want to be seen. Laurie, for example, said: "I'd like a complete physical since I haven't had one in years. I'd also like a referral for a colonoscopy because my aunt died of colon cancer in her forties. And I'd like to talk to the doctor about my changing menstrual cycle, my low back pain, and the fact that I keep getting cold sores."

Result: The office manager scheduled enough time for Laurie to have a complete physical. After the exam, the doctor talked with Laurie. He wrote the referral for the colonoscopy. He also gave her a patient handout about perimenopause and gave her a handout about an ergonomic chair and exercises she could do at her desk. Finally, he discussed the possibility of taking Zovirax as suppression therapy for cold sores. Laurie was reassured by the information on perimenopause. She bought the special chair and started doing the exercises regularly. However, she decided to forgo the medication for the cold sores unless recurrences became unbearably frequent. She was relieved, though, to know there was a recourse available should that happen.

As for Bob, he let the receptionist know he needed to talk to the doctor about his indigestion. Again, the doctor scheduled sufficient time. Bob described what he called a "heaviness" in his chest after meals. He called the sensation "heartburn." He also said he felt something in his chest when he ran to catch the commuter train. Bob then told the doctor about the pressure he was under at work, and mentioned that he was still smoking a pack a day and had put on a little weight recently. Because of all that, along with the fact that Bob's uncle had died of heart disease in his fifties, the doctor referred Bob to a cardiologist for further evaluation. The specialist dictated what is called a "consultation report" and the typed results were sent back to Bob's doctor. Bob got a copy for himself. You should do the same in a similar situation. Here is how to read the report:

Doctors typically record the notes of an office visit or consultation using a logical format referred to as "SOAP notes":

Subjective findings refer to your own complaints, symptoms, and concerns—the information you describe to the doctor.

Objective findings refer to the data your doctor collected from physical examinations and the results of any laboratory tests.

Assessment or analysis refers to the doctor's sizing up or opinion about the cause of your problem or reason for the consultation.

Plan refers to the recommendations or suggestions made by the doctor or consultant as to the best method of treatment or further testing of your condition or problem.

Bob turned out to have high cholesterol and abnormal results of a stress test. The cardiologist put Bob on a diet, exercise, and medication regimen. Bob followed it religiously, and he joined a smoking cessation program. He also managed to get transferred to a nearby branch office where the stress level was much lower. So far, he has avoided needing medication or surgery. And his "indigestion" is gone.

Now that you, like Bob and Laurie, have started your health journal and begun collecting your records and reports, keep up the good work. In the future, you can let the doctor's office know that you are returning for a follow-up either because the doctor asked to see you again or because your symptoms have persisted or gotten worse. You can also bring up new problems as they occur.

MAKE A LIST AND CHECK IT TWICE

Even though you have told the receptionist why you're scheduling an appointment, write down a list of your symptoms and questions and bring it with you. Your doctor has thousands of patient profiles to deal with. You have one. Don't assume that the receptionist or the office manager will relay all of your symptoms to the doctor, and don't expect the doctor to remember them. If he does, terrific. If he misses something and you forget or block it as well, you won't get all the care you need. Studies have shown that when patients ask questions, doctors almost always provide answers. But if you don't ask, your doctor might not tell.

Laurie says the written list worked really well for her and Bob. "I think I would have dismissed the irregular periods and the difference in the flow if I hadn't written down the facts," she says. "I'm not the kind of person who likes to dwell on my health and I don't like talking about personal stuff. But having the list made everything so much more black-and-white, not so emotional and embarrassing. I looked at it, and I was all set to speak up about what was going on with me. Bob felt exactly the same way."

You've prepared for your office visit, so let's move on to what to do when you get there.

A HAND TO HOLD

Particularly if you're feeling too sick or frightened to function well on your own behalf, bring your health buddy along. There's nothing like having a friend or relative lending support, encouraging you to tell the whole story, and helping you make sense of what the doctor says. After the visit, you'll have someone to remind you of what the doctor said, someone to make sure you follow through, someone to celebrate with if the news is good, and someone to keep your spirits up or be a shoulder to cry on if the news is bad. For a routine physical or simple screening test, you might be all right by yourself, but don't go it alone if you're worried and certainly not if a procedure will leave you groggy from a sedative. For the record, I always have someone with me and I always go with a health buddy—a special friend.

If you don't have immediate family or close friends nearby, why not call a house of worship to see whether volunteers can help you? You can also contact support groups to find a health buddy in your area. This fast-paced world can often seem indifferent and impersonal, but there really is no need to be alone and afraid. Your immune system will thank you for reaching out and connecting with someone who cares about you and who might be able to administer what really is the best medicine after all: a healthy dose of support and laughter just when you need it most.

ASK FOR COPIES OF TEST RESULTS FROM THIS VISIT, AND BRING ALONG ANY RECORDS YOU MAY ALREADY HAVE

Bob did not have any of his records in hand when he showed up for the appointment with his primary care provider. "I never had an armed services physical because I never got drafted and never enlisted. The only time I had a complete physical was when I worked for a large advertising agency that offered free exams for executive level employees," Bob says. "But I've been freelance for years now and that place I went to for the tests has gone out of business by now. It's too bad, because the exam was pretty thorough. I had an EKG, a stress test, blood work, the whole nine yards. If I had asked for my results back then, I would have something to compare with my current results. But whatever. There's nothing I can do but start from here. So I had the receptionist fax my test results." If you are in the same position as Bob is, do exactly what he did and then keep collecting your results and summaries from now on. You'll still be ahead of the game.

Laurie, like most women, had more of a history of health care than her husband did. She had given birth to two children, the first by cesarean section in a hospital and the second as a VBAC (vaginal birth after cesarean) in a birthing center staffed by midwives. She had also been seeing her gynecologist annually for pelvic, breast, and rectal exams and Pap smears. And because she served as a volunteer housemother one summer at her daughter's camp, she had a mandatory physical. "That was five years ago," she says. "I was impressed that when I called my doctor's office, they still had everything on file and sent copies right out to me when I asked for them. They wouldn't accept my offer of $15 for copying expenses. I don't know whether my experience is typical, but I was very pleased." Laurie also succeeded in getting records from her gynecologist, including her lab reports and hospital discharge summary. The birthing center, however, was no longer operating and those records were lost. Laurie filled in the gap by writing her own recollections of the circumstances surrounding the birth.

When Laurie went for her appointment with her primary care physician, she brought her written questions and her records with her but she couldn't figure out quite how to proceed. "The nurse ushered me into the examining room and told me to give a urine sample, undress, put on a gown, go sit on the examining table, and wait. I tried to picture myself balancing the file of questions and records on my lap while I was perched on the edge of the table practically naked. Maybe if my doctor had already gotten used to the system of having patients bring records, it would have been different. But as it was, I didn't think that was the moment to explain it to him. I chickened out and left my records beside my clothes. I just told him my symptoms from memory."

In the end, Laurie got a chance to share her records with her doctor and refer to her written list during a chat in his office when she was once again fully clothed. "I think that's the best plan," she says. "No matter how good the doctor is, you feel undignified during the exam. When you're dressed and sitting across from him in the office, you're human again and it's easier to be businesslike." (Note: Many doctors let you have your discussion before you put on a gown and go through the exam.)

Laurie's doctor, by the way, was impressed with her sheaf of records and encouraged her to keep up the good work. He made a note on his chart to send her a copy of the results of her blood and urine work when they arrived. She got her results in the mail two weeks later, as promised. "Maybe some doctors would resist this idea," Laurie says. "By now, though, I'm so excited about having my records that I think I would actually switch doctors if mine refused to let me in on what's happening with my own body."

EAST MEETS WEST

Important note: Bring your records whether you are visiting a traditional doctor or a complementary care provider—a category which includes Eastern medicine as well as such practitioners as chiropractors and physical therapists. Your goal is to coordinate the efforts of all your health care professionals. Don't be embarrassed to tell your doctor about your complementary therapies. Hiding information could be dangerous or simply duplicate tests and treatment.

Remember Jeremy, the hypoglycemic teenager we met back in Step 3? When his mother, Maureen, called to make an appointment for him with a nutritionist, she mentioned that she had copies of the actual blood work. The nutritionist was delighted and said that she routinely asks people to get their results for her but that a lot of people don't bother. This, of course, hinders the nutritionist in her efforts to help her clients.

Maureen made sure Jeremy's doctor knew about the dietary supplements recommended by the nutritionist. She was wise to do so. Vitamins and herbal remedies are real medicine. They can interact with prescription drugs or cause adverse reactions of their own. You have already heard me say that if you don't ask, your doctor might not tell. The second part of that message is that if you don't tell, your doctor might not ask. So help your doctor help you by speaking up about all aspects of your care.

SAY IT RIGHT

Speaking up isn't always easy, however. You don't want to come off as a self-styled know-it-all, especially if your doctor seems threatened by the new paradigm of a partnership with you. On the other hand, you may be afraid to say anything except "Yes, doctor" and "Thank you, doctor" because you have been inculcated with the idea that your doctor knows best. My suggestion is that you should practice before your office visit. Have your health buddy pretend to be your doctor while you talk about your case. Of course, the person you're rehearsing with won't know what the doctor's responses will be. That's not the issue. The point is to say things out loud in order to test how they sound, and to get over your fear of voicing concerns to your doctor.

Rule of thumb: Give your doctor symptoms (the more specific the better) but not a diagnosis (even if you think you know what's wrong). Don't say: "I'm pretty sure I have heart disease." Do say: "I've had chest pains once or twice a week for the past month and they last about ten minutes. They usually happen when I'm on the treadmill. Also, I checked my blood pressure with a home device and it's 160 over 92. I looked that up in the *Merck Manual* and it doesn't sound so good. I thought I'd better tell you what's been going on." There is nothing offensive about this manner of letting your doctor know that you are informed and aware, and that you probably have a legitimate concern. He'll be grateful for all of the information and will probably be inspired to question you further. You will have succeeded in opening up the lines of communication and creating a very productive interaction with your doctor—one which will serve the dual purpose of enhancing your chances of getting top-quality care while reducing your doctor's odds of being slapped with a malpractice suit. It's a win-win situation. Any doctor worth your time will understand that fact in an instant, and you'll come away with much more information and advice than you would have if you hadn't spoken up.

BE HONEST

Lily, a friend of mine, likes to tell the story of the time her dentist noticed that her gums were bleeding—a possible precursor of periodontal disease. The dentist asked Lily if she had been flossing regularly and she said she had. The dentist shook his head and said, "The gums don't lie." Lily blushed and admitted that she almost never flossed.

In this case, Lily's gums gave her away, but sometimes

stuff is going on internally and your doctor needs the truth about your health habits in order to help you. Don't fudge the facts or else the mystery of your health problems may not be solved in time. Maybe you don't want to admit to having one too many, but your liver knows about it anyway. Maybe the midnight food binges are your little secret, but you could be eating your way to adult onset diabetes. Your doctor is *not* going to be judgmental about your "weaknesses." Her job is to make sure you get well and stay well. Keeping anything from her only hurts you. So come clean.

MEMORIES ARE MADE OF NOTES AND TAPES

Once you have spoken up fully and forthrightly about your health, you doctor will give you feedback and advice. But his input won't do you any good if you don't remember what it is. Studies show that the average patient forgets 50 percent of what the doctor says as soon as the appointment is over. That's why you need to borrow tricks of the journalism trade, as follows:

1) Take good notes and keep them on file. Many journalists like the slim reporter's notebooks available at any stationery store. They slip easily into your briefcase or purse and can be held in the palm of one hand while you write with the other. Or, if you know shorthand, you may prefer a stenographer's notebook. Another choice would be a loose-leaf notebook, particularly if you're using the same binder to store your records. You could also bring your laptop or palmtop if that's what you're most comfortable with. The tool doesn't matter as much as the technique. Journalists (and successful college students) each develop a personal system of jotting the highlights of what they hear, and those notes trigger the whole concept when read back later on. This is an acquired skill. Practice by taking notes while

you're watching the evening news. Or have your health buddy talk to you about anything—a subject in which she's well versed, the events of her day, her problems at work. Take notes as she speaks. Then check back with her later to see how much you got right. (Bonus: If your health buddy is your spouse, this exercise may well make you more attuned to her needs and interests!)

2) Tape conversations with your doctor. Even the best notes are not infallible. If you want to capture every syllable of what your doctor says, bring a battery-operated tape recorder along when you go for office visits. You can play the tapes back later as a reminder of his instructions. You may want to transcribe the tapes and file the results with the rest of your health paperwork.

—᠊ᴧ᠊—

Interaction with your doctor doesn't end when you walk out of the office. Depending on your circumstances, you may need to contact her for booster shots of support and advice between visits. Also, an emergency may arise. Here's how to stay in touch with your doctor without imposing on her.

PHONE CALLS

When you call the doctor, take notes just as you would in the office. This minimizes the need to call back to have information repeated. Talk to your health buddy about your concerns and write down the questions in advance. You may ask your health buddy to listen to your doctor's advice with you. Let your doctor know someone else is listening.

You: "May I have my partner listen to this conversation so that I won't forget what you say?"

Your doctor: "Yes, that's fine with me."

Step 5: Helping Your Doctor Help You

Here are my guidelines for communicating with your doctor by phone:

1) Place nonemergency calls during your doctor's regular office hours only. Why annoy her by interrupting her unpaid free time asking for a prescription renewal or reporting a symptom or side effect that in all likelihood poses no immediate threat? In the case of the prescription renewal, plan ahead so you don't get caught with an empty medication bottle on a Sunday afternoon. As always, your relationship with your doctor is a two-way street. If you do your part, your doctor will be more inclined to go all out for you. That's human nature—and doctors are only human after all.

2) Absolutely any time you suspect that a situation may be an emergency, don't hesitate to pick up that phone no matter what time of night or day. Many of the symptoms on the red flag list in Step 1 warrant a call and so do any other symptoms that your instinct tells you are serious. Be prepared to communicate your sense of urgency to your doctor. Then, if he says you need to go to the emergency room, do it. (You may think that goes without saying, but it doesn't. I know from experience.)

On the other hand, if your doctor reassures you that the problem isn't critical but *you* still feel panicky, go to the ER anyway. The same is true if you leave a message with the service and the doctor or someone covering for him doesn't call back within a short time. Don't stop to worry about what the doctor will think and don't let the fact that you might not be reimbursed by the insurance company keep you from getting help. I have reviewed too many tragic malpractice cases in which people relied on the advice of a sleepy doctor who was covering for someone else and made a bad judgment call in the middle of the night. Anyway, you're the one in trouble or on the scene. You are witness-

133

ing the swelling or the bleeding. You are either feeling the pain or seeing someone grimacing and doubled over. So do call the doctor, but make the final decision based on what your "doctor within" is telling you. Certainly, as a courtesy, you can leave a message with your doctor's service about your decision to go to the ER. Any good doctor will respect your action under the circumstances, even if the problem turns out not to be serious.

E-MAIL

If both you and your doctor are into lobbing e-mail messages back and forth, this can be the perfect solution for ongoing nonemergency communication without bothering him. The advantage is that he can read his e-mail when he has the time, and respond as he sees fit. Some people worry about confidentiality, however, since nothing in cyberspace is guaranteed to be private. Even messages which have ostensibly been deleted can almost always be retrieved and used as evidence in legal situations. But if all you're doing is requesting a prescription renewal or thanking your doctor for diagnosing your problem, e-mail is an ideal medium. Warning: As is true of any means of contacting your doctor, don't overdo it. You don't want her to feel pressured to respond too often and you don't want her to think of you as a pest.

$$\downarrow\!\!\!\curvearrowleft$$

A final note: If you have established a good rapport with your doctor by following all the advice in Step 5, you'll be better able to handle the tricky business of going for a second opinion. Simply say that while you trust and respect her, you feel so nervous about your symptom or diagnosis that you'd like to have another eye on it. Of course, since you have all your own records, you could technically go to a new doctor without mentioning that to the first one. But you're far better off keeping everyone apprised of all that you're doing so that you can benefit from each expert's input. You're going to need all the cooperation and advice you can get when you take Step 6 and become involved in making choices about your own care...

Step 6 Participating in Decisions About Your Treatment Options

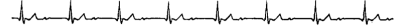

"As a man's real power grows, and his knowledge widens, ever the way he can follow grows narrower, until at last he chooses nothing, but does only and wholly what he must do."
—Ursula Le Guin in *Wizard of Earthsea*

If your appendix ruptures or you're bleeding from a gunshot wound, you are obviously not going to stop to ask questions about your care. Your only option is to trust the emergency room personnel and thank your lucky stars for the wonders of Western medicine. However, the vast majority of health problems are not the stuff of high drama. Even a frightening diagnosis such as cancer brings with it the opportunity to draw a deep breath, team up with your doctor, and figure out what the best plan of action is in your case. For just about any condition or illness, there is no one-size-fits-all solution. And studies such as the landmark Kaplan-Greenfield work show that patients who learn what their choices are and make informed decisions about how to proceed are a lot more likely to get better and feel better than are patients who don't get involved.

R_X FOR THE TAILOR-MADE TREATMENTS YOU NEED

Everything you've learned since you opened this book will come into play as you go about determining how to get the custom-made care you deserve. You need to have faith in your common sense, study your own test results and summaries, bone up on whatever your problem is, understand the purpose and conclusions of any screening or diagnostic tests, and establish a two-way relationship with your doctor.

On that last subject, however, I need to offer a note of caution. Until now, I've been writing about your doctor with the assumption that you like her. I have also assumed that no matter how overworked she may be, she is a scrupulous and compassionate person who has your best interests at heart. Most doctors, even in the current health care climate, still fit that description. Some do not. There are harrowing stories of doctors who, for their own financial gain, push patients into clinical drug trials. Also, in the medical profession as in any other, there are practitioners who aren't very good at what they do. And some doctors abuse the concept of patient involvement by simply dumping the whole responsibility for decision making in your lap without taking the time to teach you anything even if you do follow my advice about asking for information. I like to invoke the old adage that "the squeaky wheel gets the grease" when I'm encouraging people to be proactive about their health care. Most of the time, it holds true. When it doesn't, that's a very bad sign. A skilled surgeon with golden hands and an impeccable success record may not be the right doctor for you if his bedside manner leaves you cold. And even if your Aunt Betsy swears by Dr. Smith, he may not be the one for you if you're not comfortable talking with him. The unfathomable mystery of what makes people click with each other applies to your relationship with your doctor just as it does with anyone else.

Beyond the realm of the personal, keep in mind that generations of American physicians have been trained to treat aggressively. Also, a fear of malpractice suits makes doctors want to be able to say "I did all I could." The result is a situation in which you may be railroaded into taking powerful medication or undergoing surgery when a less drastic watch-and-wait option involving lifestyle changes might work just as well or better. Consider the fact that more than one third of patients on the list for heart transplants at the University of California in Los Angeles improved so much with personalized exercise programs and simple diuretics that they didn't need new hearts after all. And an inflammation which commonly causes kidney failure has been shown to go into spontaneous remission or disappear altogether in a full 60 percent of patients who refuse the standard treatment of steroids and immune suppressers. Also, for the majority of men with a condition called benign prostatic hypertrophy (BPH), surgery is no sure cure and occasionally causes complications such as impotence or incontinence. Simple monitoring may be all that's called for; or at most, a medication to relieve nuisance symptoms such as frequent or painful urination.

As a doctor, I have to admit that it's not always easy to let patients choose a conservative approach, but that is ultimately what should be done if a patient is fully informed and capable of making a decision. I remember Martha, an African-American woman in her sixties who had a very large abdominal aneurysm—a bulge in a blood vessel that is almost certainly fatal if it ruptures. I recommended bypass surgery, since her aneurysm was two centimeters above the danger level. I believed with all my heart that this was the right way to go, particularly since her race was an added risk factor. She didn't agree. She brought her husband and her sister in to talk with me about other options, and she let me know that her religious faith was very strong. I worked with her until we devised a diet, exercise, and medication regimen designed to lower her blood pressure just enough but not too much, given her condition. As I always do when I prescribe medication, I explained exactly what was wrong with the patient and how the medication could treat the problem. I also gave instructions about how to take the medication. Before beginning any medication, make sure your doctor does the same for you, and always ask these questions:

1) What is the name of the medication?

2) Is that a brand name? If so, is the cheaper generic version just as good? (It isn't always.)

3) Is this drug from my approved managed care formulary? If yes, would I be better off with an alternative drug that is not covered by my insurance?

4) What is the purpose of this medication and why does it make sense for my condition?

5) What good effect will probably result from my taking the medicine?

6) What side effects, if any, might I experience? Is there any way to alleviate them?

7) What will happen to my health if I decide not to take the medicine?

8) What is the starting dose?

9) How long and how often should I take the medicine?

10) Are there any special instructions, such as taking the medicine with food or on an empty stomach?

11) Can I drink alcoholic beverages while I'm taking the medicine?

12) Will this medicine interact with any of the other drugs I am taking?

13) What should I do if I forget to take a pill? Should I just skip that dose or take a double dose next time?

14) Is it safe to stop taking the medicine abruptly? Why or why not?

15) How will I know the medicine is working? What is my goal? (For example, LDL cholesterol under 100 or blood pressure [BP] under 120/80.)

16) What is the maximum amount of this pill that can safely be taken daily?

I went over those sixteen questions with Martha, the sixty-ish woman with the large aneurysm. She was highly motivated to succeed with her medication regimen and she followed my instructions to the letter. Her blood pressure went down and she lived for five more years that I know of before she retired to Florida—hopefully to enjoy a ripe old age.

This story demonstrates that in the best of all possible worlds, you would have a doctor who respected your wishes and did everything possible to give you the information you needed to weigh your options. He would have you look at the risks and benefits of each possibility in light of your family health history, your values, your own health history, and your lifestyle. Such a doctor also would not give up on you if you rejected a recommendation for aggressive treatment. He would go the distance with you in trying a conservative route. And he would listen if you changed your mind at any point, and help you explore alternatives.

To find out how a scenario such as that would work, let's play a guessing game. I'm going to explain the risks and benefits of hormone replacement therapy (HRT) for menopausal women. In order to do this, I'll give you the profiles of two very different women who were my patients. Incidentally, both of these women asked me a typical question: "What would you do yourself, doctor?" Male physicians tell me that the version of this question which they hear is: "What would you have your wife do, doctor?" Unfortunately, as you will see, each case is so individual that there is no blanket solution. What is right for me or for a male doctor's wife might not be right for you. This is the art, not the science, of medicine with which we're dealing. To understand what I mean, follow along as I take you through the way I worked with Ginger and Barbara. Try to figure out which option each woman chose, based on all the relevant factors. Then I'll let you in on what really happened.

A TALE OF TWO PATIENTS

Barbara was forty-nine when she first started missing periods and experiencing hot flashes. Ginger, another patient, was fifty-one when she called to say she thought she might be going into menopause. Both of these women had heard about HRT. As Barbara put it: "It seems like all of my friends take estrogen. Isn't that what women are supposed to do?"

Not necessarily. Back in the 1960s and early 1970s, the answer would have been yes, but we have learned a lot since the days of giving doses of estrogen which were ten times higher than we now recommend. And back then, the estrogen was "unopposed," meaning that it was not prescribed in combination with progesterone. Not only that, but we prescribed the estrogen replacement therapy (ERT) to virtually all women who asked for (and could afford) this perceived Fountain of Youth. The result was that of the women who took ERT, there was a four- to tenfold increase in the risk of uterine cancer. After that scare, research was done in earnest to come up with better options, and studies were also done to find out whether HRT could have long-term *positive* effects on women's health. In the 1980s, research showed that HRT could protect women's bones. In the 1990s we learned that HRT could protect women against heart disease. Consequently, HRT today serves as a perfect example of how important it is for you to look at a balance sheet and participate in your own health care decisions.

To start with, I'm going to tell you what I discussed with Barbara and Ginger about the two reasons for considering HRT. The first is symptomatic relief. During the two or three years when women are going through the infamous "change," many of them are uncomfortable and some are downright miserable. Barbara was in the latter number. "I haven't had a full night's sleep in months," she said. "I wake up hot and sweaty two or three times at least. I've started camping out on the sofabed. It's not fair for Harry to end up sleep-deprived, too. Sometimes I'm soaked and have to change the sheets and my nightgown. I can't go on much longer like this. I'm turning into a witch with a capital B and I can't concentrate at work anymore. Help!"

Barbara also said that her daytime hot flashes were embarrassing and demoralizing. "My face turns red and my makeup runs. I've started wearing dress shields. But what I really hate is that the hot flashes are reminders that I'm getting old. I look in the mirror and see this beet-red person who is running out of estrogen, which translates into running out of time."

That is one woman's experience. Ginger had another story to tell. "This is no big deal," she said. "I have hot flashes every once in a while but nobody would know it, and I only wake up at night every now and then. I kind of like the hot flashes, actually. It's an interesting sensation, not at all like breaking a sweat when you're exercising. The heat comes from inside and there's a little rush when it happens. I think a woman's body is a miracle. This is just another stage in that miracle—menstruation, pregnancy, labor and delivery, breastfeeding, and then the natural end of the childbearing years. Besides, I keep thinking about how great it will be when this is over in a little while and I won't have to bother with my periods or worry about getting pregnant. My husband never had a vasectomy and I never had a tubal, so this will be our first chance in twenty-five years to make love without birth control. What a way to celebrate our Silver Anniversary!"

Obviously, Barbara and Ginger were on the opposite ends of the scale when it came to experiencing menopausal symptoms. However, I outlined the symptomatic relief HRT could provide.

1) Hot Flashes HRT stops the hot flashes, unequivocally. The flashes will subside on their own after a couple of years, but Barbara's face lit up when she heard that she wouldn't have to wait it out. She was also glad to hear that contrary to a prevailing myth, HRT does not put hot flashes "on hold." If a woman stops taking HRT for some reason after the time when nature would have run its course, the hot flashes won't start up again. Ginger just shrugged when she heard all of this. She was clearly not interested.

2) Aches and Pains This vague category of postmenopausal complaints has only anecdotal evidence to support the relief HRT might bring. For Barbara, who suffered from low back and knee pain plus general stiffness in the morning, the potential relief was a possible bonus of the therapy. Ginger, though, said she felt as fit as ever. She also had a firm belief that menopause is not a disease but a natural process women are meant to go through. She felt that there is no need to "medicalize" it.

—ᴧᴧ—

But as I said, symptomatic relief is only one reason to take HRT. The second is prevention. HRT is believed to protect women from certain diseases. Here is the list of possible benefits of HRT which I shared with Barbara and Ginger:

1) **Heart Disease** Young women are much less likely than men to succumb to heart disease. But statistics show that after menopause, women lose their edge. Taking estrogen may correct for that. There is good evidence that estrogen improves the lipid profile (see page 86), meaning that it lowers levels of "bad cholesterol" while raising levels of "good cholesterol." In addition, the estrogen smooths out the lining of the arteries, making the blood vessels more resilient.

After I explained this to Barbara and Ginger, I reviewed with them their personal risk factors. First, I asked each of them whether they had close male relatives who had died of heart disease under the age of fifty-five and/or close female relatives who had died of heart disease under the age of sixty-five. Barbara, who came from German and Swedish stock, said no. But Ginger said that her father, a Mexican-American, had died of a heart attack at the age of forty-six. Statistically, people of Hispanic descent and African-Americans are at higher than average risk for complications of heart disease. I told Ginger to make a note of that. I had already asked both women to keep a running tally of pluses and minuses on our way to making a decision about HRT.

Then I looked at other factors. Ginger had quit smoking twenty years earlier. Her weight was only a few pounds above what it had been in her salad days. She belonged to a gym, her blood pressure was normal, and she didn't have diabetes. However, her total cholesterol was 50 points higher than the reference range, her "good cholesterol" was too low, and her "bad cholesterol" was too high.

Barbara didn't have diabetes, but she did have high cholesterol and mild hypertension. She was a buxom beauty who had always been about thirty pounds overweight, and she was a two-pack-a-day smoker. By her own admission, she was a confirmed couch potato.

2) Osteoporosis Bony resorption is a continual remodeling process in which the body gets rid of used bone before replacing it with new. Osteoporosis is a disease in which the loss of old bony material happens faster than the rebuilding. The result is a decrease in the density of the bone mass and with it an increased risk of fractures, particularly of the wrist, spine, and hips. Advanced cases can involve the stooped "Dowager's hump" and painful "crush fractures" of the spine that occur simply from the effort of standing up. Postmenopausal women are prone to osteoporosis because when estrogen production stops, bony resorption increases. Studies have shown that the resulting loss of density can be rapid during the first five years after menopause. For some women, a calcium-rich diet and calcium supplements plus regular weight-bearing exercise are sufficient to help keep that loss at a minimum. For other women, HRT provides essential extra protection, cutting in half the risk of fractures of the hip and reducing by a whopping 90 percent the risk of fractures of the spine.

I talked with Barbara and Ginger to see which category each of them fell into. Neither one was on bone-robbing steroids or thyroid medication. However, Barbara's sedentary lifestyle was a strike against her. So was the fact that every day she had two martinis at the Happy Hour followed by wine with dinner and a cognac afterward. Her smoking wasn't helping either, and incidentally, it was almost certainly one of the reasons she was going into menopause earlier than the average woman. The one thing Barbara had going for her was her zaftig figure. The extra pounds weren't doing her heart any good, but her bones were benefiting from the weight. There was a fair chance that like her mother and grandmother before her—both of them ample-bodied women—Barbara wouldn't develop osteoporosis. And in fact, a DEXA scan, the virtually surefire test to diagnose osteoporosis (see page 100), showed that Barbara still had normal spinal bone density of T + 1.

Ginger hadn't been as lucky as Barbara. Her DEXA scan showed the beginnings of spinal bone loss, a condition called osteopenia. Her T-score was -1.8. I wasn't surprised. Ginger had gotten her nickname early on because of her red hair, but she had gone gray in her late twenties just as her Irish-born mother had. The red hair, the premature gray, and the Northern European blood were all tip-offs that Ginger was a candidate for bone loss. Ginger also got her fair and freckled skin—another sign of predisposition to osteoporosis—from the O'Connor side of the family, and she told me that one of her maternal aunts had broken her hip when she was in her seventies. As for other factors, Ginger was trim but not small-boned, which was a plus. Her regular exercise was helping her as well. On the negative side, her diet contained only about 600 milligrams of calcium because she didn't like milk and had heard it was bad for her cholesterol. The fact that she had quit smoking was in her favor, however, as was her pattern of drinking no more than a couple of glasses of wine a few times a week.

3) Alzheimer's Disease Several research projects including the Baltimore Study on Aging have turned up preliminary evidence that HRT may help prevent or slow down the tragic loss of memory that characterizes Alzheimer's. This disorder strikes about 10 percent of the population in the last third of life. Although it may be hereditary, there is no conclusive genetic link, so a family history or lack thereof isn't a good predictor one way or another. Lifestyle factors aren't clearly implicated either. In other words, there's no way to evaluate whether you're at risk. Still, I wanted both Barbara and Ginger to know about the possible protection against Alzheimer's which HRT may afford.

4) **Colon Cancer** The Nurses' Study in Boston showed that HRT may help ward off cancer of the colon and/or rectum. Neither Barbara nor Ginger had a family history of the disease. Given their ages, I suggested they should schedule colonoscopies or at the very least, do stool checks or schedule sigmoidoscopies (see pages 89–93). Barbara's diet, rich in the fats and sugars she enjoyed so much, probably did put her at some risk. Ginger, the fish/whole grains/vegetable fanatic, was statistically less likely to develop colon cancer.

By this time, Barbara and Ginger had a list of possible benefits of HRT and the beginnings of a personal profile. We moved on to the risks of HRT:

1) **Breast Cancer** The Nurses' Study in Boston suggested that HRT slightly increases the risk of getting cancer of the breast after five years of being on the medication. There is speculation that the HRT does not cause the cancer but simply fuels and speeds up a cancer that was already there.

Barbara squirmed in her seat when I told her that. Her mother, her grandmother, and her mother's sister had all died of breast cancer in their forties. At forty-nine, Barbara had been spared so far but with a family history like that, she feared she might be a time bomb.

Ginger had no family history of breast cancer. I recommended that they both schedule a baseline mammogram and have one yearly after that. They agreed to do so.

2) **Uterine Cancer** With today's HRT, the risk of this form of cancer is extremely slight. We rarely prescribe "unopposed" estrogen to women who have not had hysterec-

tomies. Instead, we team the estrogen with progesterone. That greatly reduces the chance of a buildup of the lining of the uterus which could go on to become cancer. Still, women like Barbara who are overweight tend to have extra circulating estrogen after menopause. The estrogen is produced by fat cells and can lead to endometrial hyperplasia (buildup of the lining of the uterus). For Ginger, lithe and slim, that wasn't likely to be a problem.

3) **Phlebitis** This is a condition in which blood clots form in the veins. The clots can travel to the lungs with serious and sometimes fatal consequences. HRT slightly increases the risk of this condition. By the way, so does Evista, the new so-called designer estrogen. Evista, a synthetic, has only been on the market for five years, while estrogen has been around for decades. Yet to my amazement, women have rushed to get Evista. My advice is to proceed with caution until we know much more about the long-term effects of Evista. In any case, women with a history of phlebitis should not take HRT or Evista, and all women who take HRT need to stop the therapy a few weeks before elective surgery. For both Barbara and Ginger, there was no history of phlebitis.

4) **Gallstones** There is a slight increase in the incidence of gallstones in women who take HRT. Neither Barbara nor Ginger had ever had symptoms of this disorder, but Barbara's liver function results (see page 85), showed that she was somewhat out of range, probably because of the dry martinis, the fine wines, and the cognacs she loved so much.

5) **Migraines** Many women who suffer from migraines report that attacks are less frequent or disappear altogether after menopause. Some women with a history of migraines say the attacks get worse on HRT. Barbara and Ginger had never had migraines.

6) **Weight Gain and Bloating** Some women say they feel as though they're in a different body on HRT. However, virtually all women tend to gain some weight after menopause whether they are on HRT or not. This may be nature's way of protecting against osteoporosis. Barbara didn't care much about the possible weight gain on HRT, but Ginger recoiled at the thought of her body changing. I reminded her that if she started the therapy and hated the way she felt, she could choose to stop after a trial of a month or two.

The lists were complete. Barbara and Ginger each took a couple of days to look them over and discuss them with friends and family to get some perspective. They also did some research on their own. Now comes your chance to guess what each woman decided. Go back over the previous pages and put yourself in Barbara's shoes, then in Ginger's shoes. What do you think they did?

Here are the answers. Barbara, who had been so eager for symptomatic relief, chose to give up that short-term benefit rather than increase her already great risk of getting breast cancer. Of course this meant she had to pass up the protective power of HRT against heart disease, Alzheimer's, and colon cancer. Even so, I agreed with her decision and applauded her for making a difficult choice. I reminded her that there were many ways she could help herself. After reviewing the profile which emerged during our decision-making process, she was motivated for the first time in her life to take better care of her health. I helped her make a phase-by-phase plan so that changing her ways wouldn't seem overwhelming. When we get to Step 8, you'll follow Barbara as she manages to lose weight, start exercising, quit smoking, and stop drinking. Also in Step 8, you'll learn how she weighed the pros and cons of a controversial prophy-lactic procedure to prevent breast cancer.

For now, let me just give you the good news about how she fared during and after menopause without HRT. The lifestyle modifications got Barbara's blood pressure down to near normal levels, but we decided she should also be tak-ing a mild diuretic. The diuretic causes the body to lose extra fluids for a couple of weeks, but the main purpose is to lower the blood pressure. I also put her on a low-salt diet and advised her to eat oranges and bananas to guard against potassium loss from the diuretic. I had her take 1,200 mil-ligrams of calcium a day, and a multivitamin without iron but with folic acid to reduce the risk of heart disease and colon cancer. As of this writing, she feels better than she has in years and years—and the hot flashes and joint pain are long since behind her.

What about Ginger? She began our decision-making process dead set against tampering with menopause, which she saw as a normal course of events. Certainly, she had no desire to go on HRT for symptomatic relief only. After all, her symptoms were minimal, probably due in part to her admirable attitude and health habits. Yet Ginger did elect to take HRT. The family history on her father's side for early heart disease and on her mother's side for osteoporosis were the deciding factors for her. There's a cynical joke that goes: "Eat right, exercise, die anyway." But it was not a laughing matter for Ginger. No amount of clean living was going to guarantee that she could fend off the problems she was prone to by virtue of her genes. The solution Ginger and I came up with was to put her on oral estrogen rather than the patch, because the oral version would be more likely to benefit her cholesterol. I put her on 1,200 milligrams of cal-cium, 400 units of vitamin D, and a multivitamin without iron. I did not prescribe a cholesterol-lowering drug nor a drug to slow down bony resorption. I felt that a trial with just the HRT was in order and Ginger and I discussed the pros and cons of all these decisions.

Ginger remained apprehensive about gaining weight on the HRT, but she agreed to give it a try. After two months, she came back for a checkup extremely pleased. She had kept up her exercise and hadn't gained any weight or gotten puffy. She said her hot flashes were gone and that she was sleeping soundly. She was surprised how much better that made her feel even though she had insisted earlier that she hadn't minded the hot flashes. Ginger also liked the idea that she might be saving herself from Alzheimer's and might even be sharpening her cognitive powers a bit. As for breast cancer, she understood that her risk was slightly increased but she decided to take the chance given everything else she had to consider. She simply resolved to be religious about regular screening tests (see page 111).

Did you guess the actual outcomes? If not, you didn't lose our game. Shared and informed decision making is always a win-win situation. What made sense to Barbara or Ginger might not make sense to you. Maybe the risk of breast cancer would scare you off of HRT no matter what. Or maybe the symptomatic relief is so important to you that you'd take the HRT at least for a few years just so you wouldn't be incapacitated. It's your life and it's your body. Ideally your doctor would avoid dictating to you, or even pressuring you. He would give you a complete picture so that you could go into any treatment scenario with your eyes wide open and your expectations realistic. As for you, you would pay close attention to the information you were given, remembering that there is no such thing as a dumb question. You would then put a great deal of thought into making your choice. And you wouldn't forget to consult with your health buddy before going back to your doctor to discuss your decision.

This kind of interaction between you and your doctor works for any situation in which choices are possible. Men with prostate problems, patients weighing the pros and cons of various cancer therapies, people who have to manage asthma and diabetes, anyone facing elective surgery—all of these people will vastly improve their chances of doing well if they are an integral part of the decisions about their care. The simple reason is that they will feel in control. When we feel helpless and buffeted by forces outside of ourselves, our brains and bodies go into alert mode. As has often been said, that's great if you're about to run away from a tiger. But the willy-nilly endocrine activity that comes with the "fight or flee" response plays havoc with your immune system when it has no outlet. On the other hand, knowing that you are ultimately in charge of choosing how to deal with your health problems puts you back in the emotional driver's seat. That's the only place to be if you want to save your own life.

I know what you're thinking. Being in control is one thing when you're still going about your daily life, even if you've been diagnosed with something scary. But how do you hang on to your autonomy and dignity when you find yourself in a hospital bed, at the mercy of the staff members who breeze in and out of your room while you lie there tethered to an IV? Come on along to Step 7, and I'll let you in on some secrets from behind the scenes. Remember, I was a nurse before I was a doctor. I've never forgotten what I learned back then...

Step 7 Knowing How to Get the Best Care in the Hospital

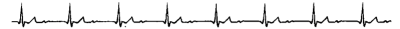

> "It may seem a strange principle to enunciate as the
> very first requirement in a Hospital that it should
> do the sick no harm."
> —Florence Nightingale

Donna went pale when she heard her mother's voice on the phone, weak and raspy. "I hate to worry you," her mother said. "I know how busy you are. I'm in the hospital. Carla came to clean today, and she insisted on driving me here. I guess I looked pretty bad. I have a terrible stomachache." Without missing a beat, Donna said, "I'll catch the next plane out. I'll be there before you know it." Her mother, eighty-five and fiercely independent, protested. But Donna knew that something was very wrong and that she needed to get from Chicago to Cleveland as soon as possible. "Jake can take care of the kids," Donna said firmly. "I'll call the school and have them get me a sub. No problem. See you soon. Love you lots!" And she was on her way.

Within hours, Donna was at her mother's bedside. Dr. Jenks, who had taken care of the family for years, was not there. A doctor called a "hospitalist" was in charge. Her mother was scheduled for an abdominal CAT scan the next morning. Nobody was saying anything about what the diagnosis might be. An aide came in with a dinner tray, but Donna's mother shook her head and wouldn't touch the food. It crossed Donna's mind that her mother probably shouldn't have been eating anyway before the CAT scan, but Donna didn't have the nerve to say anything right then to the nurse. Donna's mother dozed off, and Donna left quietly.

She drove the rental car back to her girlhood home. Her mother had been living there alone since Donna's father died ten years earlier. The place was as tidy as ever and smelled of her mother's perfume. Donna called her brother in California, and broke down in tears when she told him what was going on. "Mama looked so tiny in that hospital bed, all hooked up to tubes and stuff," Donna sobbed. "I just had this weird feeling about leaving her there alone." And that's when a realization hit Donna like a cartoon light bulb over her head. She hadn't made the trip from Chicago to Cleveland just to sit in the house. She might as well not have come if she wasn't going to be there for her mother night and day. "Will they let me stay with her?" she asked her brother. "There's only one way to find out," he said. With that, Donna went back to the hospital. Visiting hours were over, but she spoke to the head nurse and pleaded her case. The nurse agreed that Donna could sleep in the recliner in her mother's room. "I'm going to be your private duty nurse," Donna said, and her mother gave her a weak little smile.

Donna's mother was diagnosed with severe diverticulitis, an infection of the pouches in the wall of the colon, which could rupture and require surgery. She was put on intravenous antibiotics. In the days that followed, Donna was amazed at how much she was needed. When she had gotten to know the staff, she asked about whether her mother should have been given dinner on the night before the CAT scan. The answer was that the tray had been brought by mistake. From then on, Donna checked all the orders and politely asked about anything that seemed amiss. Once, when Donna had gone down to the cafeteria for lunch, her mother wanted the bedpan but couldn't reach the buzzer to call for help. After that, Donna literally never left the room except to go buy some food for herself and bring it right back. She called the nurse when the IV was running dry, she buzzed when her mother started coughing and gagging, she helped the aides bathe and turn her mother regularly, she gently asked the staff to call her mother "Mrs. Whitmire" instead of "Granny," and she mentioned that there was no need to shout since her mother had not gone deaf. Donna also asked questions and studied her mother's chart. She was careful not to seem pushy, and the staff grew quite fond of her.

Yet Donna wasn't only acting as a kind of unofficial nurse's aide. She was there in her role as a loving daughter. She read to her mother and they laughed about good times past. She also soothed her mother when the woman in the next bed started moaning. In fact, she helped the other woman as well simply by talking with her in a friendly way and making her feel less frightened. Magically, the moaning subsided and the woman fell asleep.

Within less than a week, Donna's mother was ready to go home. Donna and her mother were both thrilled that the problem hadn't turned out to be immediately life-threatening. But they were comforted nonetheless by the fact that they had been prepared with a living will and that Donna had durable power of attorney for health care for her mother. If the news had not been good, Donna's mother would have had her wishes respected regarding such issues as life support and resuscitation, and Donna could have spoken for her mother if that had been necessary. Fortunately, that sad scenario didn't play out.

Donna says she will be forever grateful that she was able

to keep her mother's hospital stay from being an impersonal and scary saga. Instead, it became a time for caring, sharing, and growing closer than they had ever been before.

SOMEONE TO WATCH OVER YOU

This is the nurse in me talking: Do what Donna did if someone you love is hospitalized. While I was at my father's bedside after his heart surgery, I not only helped with every little thing but I had the chance to hear him spin some yarns from his boyhood and listen to his opinions on things I never even knew he had been thinking about. When a life is at stake or even if someone is simply very ill, pettiness and mundane problems fade away. People's emotions become keener. Lights seem brighter. Sounds seem sweeter. The words we sometimes forget to say or find hard to say—simple ones like "Thanks for everything" and "I love you"—suddenly come easily. Don't miss the opportunities that a round-the-clock hospital vigil can bring for bonding with someone you care about.

By the same token, don't be embarrassed to get someone to stay with you if you're the patient. Thirty years ago when I was still an RN, that would have been good advice. Today, it's the *only* way to be safe and get the care you need. I remember what it was like to tend to the needs of a wardful of patients, some of them desperately ill, and I remember wishing that many of them could be monitored around the clock. But at least my colleagues and I were registered nurses. Now, with RNs in short supply and cost-cutting a top priority, you have no guarantee that a nurse will be the one who responds to your buzzer. When you need help in the middle of the night, the person who comes in may be a licensed practical nurse (LPN) or a licensed vocational nurse (LVN) who has studied for two years at a community college. You may even get a volunteer or an aide who has no formal medical education. When you're sick and possibly groggy from medication, you're not in a position to judge whether you're getting the care you need. It is essential to have an alert health buddy on hand who can assess the situation and insist that a qualified person have a look at you if that seems warranted. A few enlightened hospitals are already encouraging this practice, using the term "care partner" for the family member or friend who joins the health care team. Other hospitals, as Donna's experience demonstrates, will let you stay if you ask. So ask.

What I'm saying is that we could take up this whole chapter bemoaning the sorry state of hospital care in this country, but what good would that do? We could shake our heads over any number of statistics and horror stories about nurses accidentally giving lethal overdoses of medication, technicians failing to monitor vital signs that point to imminent respiratory failure, and surgeons amputating the wrong limbs. But that wouldn't solve anything. Let's just accept for the moment that the system is a mess. There aren't enough nurses. Untrained people are doing tasks that shouldn't be trusted to them. Residents are bleary with fatigue. Young doctors serving as "night floats" haven't got a clue about the history and status of the patients they're seeing. Hospitalists who are not familiar with patients' cases are taking over from family doctors. Many hospitals are so huge and sprawling that a design element called "wayfinding" has been devised involving color coding and maps to keep sick and confused people from getting lost. And insurance companies have hospital stays pared down to a harrowing minimum.

Those are the facts. Yes, I'd love to be instrumental in changing the system for the better. But in the meantime, let's be practical. Having a health buddy at your hospital bedside twenty-four hours a day is the way to work with the system as it stands now. I believe this is true whether or not you can afford an expensive private duty nurse. Your health buddy probably doesn't have a professional health care background, but love is very good medicine, as Donna's story shows. The value and comfort of having someone close by who is dear to you far outweighs the need for specialized knowledge. Anyway, nobody at any price cares as much as you do about your own.

As I said, I have practiced what I preach. My sister and my mother and I took turns staying with my father while he was in the hospital for heart bypass surgery. And when my husband was admitted with a potentially fatal aortic aneurysm, I made arrangements for another doctor to cover my practice. Luckily, our three young sons had just left for their first summer at sleep-away camp. However, I would have gotten someone to stay with them if necessary. I spent a full two weeks bivouacked at Brad's side. Incidentally, almost nothing that I did during that time tapped into my medical expertise. I was not there in my capacity as a physician. Far from it. I was there to notice when he needed his sheets changed after a drenching sweat. I got him water, I helped the aides bathe him, I went with him to the X-ray room to cheer him and keep track of him during the long wait for his turn, I emptied the urinal, I held damp towels to his brow when his fever was high, and I politely kept well-meaning visitors from staying too long and wearing him out. Also, as I had with my father, I listened with the kind of undivided attention we seldom give one another in this fast-paced world. Our marriage, not to mention life itself, has been more precious to both of us since then.

However, there is one way in which my medical training was an advantage while I was acting as my husband's health buddy. I knew what the abbreviations on Brad's chart meant, and therefore I could understand what was being noted about his progress. So that you can have that same advantage, here's a list of the most commonly used abbreviations and symbols. (Tip: Bring a notebook or legal pad and make your own progress notes. You can also leave a note with questions for the doctor taped to the door of the room if you are running down to the cafeteria for a minute or a whole meal.)

WHAT YOUR CHART REALLY SAYS

ADL   usual daily activities such as eating, dressing, walking (activities of daily living)

AMA   refusing reasonable and necessary medical treatment despite urging from your doctor, against medical advice

ASA   aspirin; acetylsalicylic acid

ASAP   as soon as possible, urgent

ASCVD   atherosclerotic cardiovascular disease (heart disease from hardening of the arteries to the heart leading to angina or heart attack); same as ASHD and CAD

ASHD   arteriosclerotic heart disease; same as ASCVD and CAD

BE   barium enema: X-ray dye test of the large colon

BID	twice daily
BKA	below knee amputation; amputation below the knee
BP	blood pressure
BPH	benign prostatic hypertrophy (enlarged prostate—common in older men)
BUN	blood urea nitrogen (a blood chemistry test of kidney function)
Bx	biopsy
c̄	with
C1	first cervical vertebra
Ca, CA	carcinoma (cancer); calcium
CAD	coronary artery disease (same as ASCVD and ASHD)
CBC	blood test for complete blood count
CHD	coronary heart disease (same as ASCVD, ASHD, and CAD)
CHF	congestive heart failure
Chol	cholesterol

CN   cranial nerve (peripheral nerves' origination in brainstem area)

CNS   central nervous system

COPD   chronic obstructive pulmonary disease; emphysema

Cor   heart

CRF   chronic renal (kidney) failure

C&S   culture and sensitivity (culture to look for bacteria causing an infection and find out what antibiotics can treat it)

C-sect. cesarean section

CV   cardiovascular

CVA   cerebrovascular accident (stroke); costovertebral angle (midback or flank area overlying kidneys)

Cx   cervix; culture

CXR   chest X-ray

D&C   dilation and curettage (scraping of the inside of the uterus or womb in a woman with abnormal bleeding to find the cause)

d/c, /DC, D/C discontinue, discharge from hospital or care

DDx   differential diagnosis (a list of possible causes or diagnoses for symptoms)

DIFF   differential blood count (a test of the number and types of white blood cells in the blood)

DM   diabetes mellitus (IDDM=insulin dependent diabetes mellitus or Type I; AODM=adult onset diabetes mellitus, not insulin dependent, or Type II)

DOE   dyspnea on exertion (shortness of breath on walking or going up stairs or incline)

DTR   deep tendon reflexes (e.g., knee-jerk response when doctor taps knee with hammer)

DVT   deep vein thrombosis; phlebitis or blood clots in the vein

Dx   diagnosis

EBL   estimated blood loss, commonly reported during any surgery

EEG   electroencephalogram; brain wave test

EKG, ECG   electrocardiogram; test of heart electrical activity

ENT   ear, nose, throat

EOM   extraocular movement (eye movement)

ESR   erythrocyte sedimentation rate (a test that gives a rough measure of inflammation or infection)

ETOH   alcohol

E+OH   alcoholic

FBS   fasting blood sugar (measuring blood sugar or glucose after an overnight fast)

Fe   iron

F/U   follow-up; future appointment, testing, or treatment needed

GI   gastrointestinal

GM, gm   gram, a metric measure of weight

h   hour

HBP   high blood pressure

Hct   hematocrit (blood count); test for anemia or percentage of red blood cells

HEENT   head, eyes, ears, nose, throat

Hgb, Hb   hemoglobin (measures amount of oxygen-carrying protein on the red blood cells, test for anemia)

H/H   hemoglobin and hematocrit; most common tests for anemia are often reported together

H/O   history of

H&P   history and physical; written report by your doctor describing your medical history and physical examination

HPI   history of present illness; description of your current symptoms or complaints

HS, hs   bedtime (hour of sleep)

HSV   herpes simplex virus (Type I causes fever blisters; Type II causes genital ulcers)

HTN   hypertension (high blood pressure)

Hx   history

ICU   intensive care unit

I&D   incision and drainage (e.g., lancing of an abscess or boil)

IM   intramuscular (an injection of medication or vaccine directly into the muscle)

I&O   intake and output; a measurement of all your fluid intake (by intravenous and by mouth) as well as all your urine and other liquid output such as vomiting material

IV   intravenous

IVP intravenous pyelogram (kidney dye X-ray)

JVP jugular venous pressure (visible measure of the jugular vein pressure in the neck; if elevated, a sign of heart failure)

L2, L3 second, third lumbar vertebra

LBP low back pain

LLE left lower extremity (left leg)

LLQ left lower quadrant of the abdomen

LMP last menstrual period

LNMP last normal menstrual period

LUE left upper extremity (left arm)

LV left ventricle (the largest muscle or chamber of the heart that pumps blood into the aorta)

LVH left ventricular hypertrophy (thickening of the left ventricle muscle, typically from untreated high blood pressure)

'lytes common blood electrolytes (Na—sodium, K—potassium, Cl—chloride, Co_2—carbon dioxide)

M murmurs

MCP   metacarpophalangeal joints (the joints between hand and fingers)

meq   milliequivalents (a metric unit of measurement)

MI   myocardial infarction, mitral valve leakage or insufficiency

MOM   milk of magnesia

MTP   metatarsophalangeal joints (the joints between foot and toes)

Na   sodium; blood electrolyte

NAD   no acute distress; no severe distress or discomfort

NG   nasogastric; tube through the nose to the stomach or gastric area

NKA/ NKDA   no known drug allergies

NL, nl   normal

NPO   nothing by mouth; not eating or drinking anything (as before or after surgery)

NSR   normal sinus or heart rhythm; same as RSR

N&V   nausea and vomiting

O: objective; doctor's description of physical and laboratory exam findings

$\bar{o}$ no or nothing

O2   oxygen

OBS   organic brain syndrome; confusion, senility

OD   right eye

O&P   ova and parasites; commonly checked for in the stool of person with diarrhea

OR   operating room

OS   left eye

OTC   over-the-counter (medications sold without a prescription)

OU   both eyes

$\bar{p}$ after

P   pulse or number of pulse or heart beats in a minute

pc   after meal

PCN   penicillin

PE   pulmonary embolism or physical examination findings

PERRLA   pupils, equal, round, reactive to light and accommodation (far and near vision)

PFT   pulmonary function test

PMH   past medical history

PND   paroxysmal nocturnal dyspnea (waking up at night short of breath, seen with heart failure)

PO, po   by mouth

PPD   purified protein derivative (skin test for tuberculosis)

ppd   refers to number of packs of cigarettes smoked daily, e.g., 1 ppd (1 pack per day)

pre-op   before surgery

PRN   as the occasion or need requires

PT   physical therapy; prothrombin time (a test of blood clotting, measure of the blood-thinning effect of Coumadin)

pt   patient

PTT   partial thromboplastin time (a test of blood clotting, measure of the blood-thinning effect of heparin)

PUD   peptic ulcer disease; stomach or duodenal ulcer

q   every

q4h   every four hours

qd   once a day

qh   every hour

qid   four times daily

RBC   red blood cell

R/O   rule out; differential diagnosis considerations or possibilities

ROM   range of motion; maximum movement of a joint in all possible directions

ROS   review of systems (review of all your symptoms and concerns from head to toe)

RSR   regular sinus rhythm; same as NSR

RTC   return to clinic; date when advised to return to doctor's office for appointment

RUQ   right upper quadrant of the abdomen; overlying liver and gallbladder

Rx   prescription; treatment

S   subjective; description of your symptoms or complaints by your doctor

s   without

S1   first heart sound made by closure of your mitral valve

S2   second heart sound made by closure of your aortic valve

SH   social history such as occupation, cigarette and alcohol use, family support

SMA   sequential multiple analyzer (blood chemistry check of multiple tests)

SOB   shortness of breath

S/P, s/p status post (after or previous history of a surgery or medical condition)

STD   sexually transmitted disease such as herpes, syphilis, gonorrhea

T4   thyroid hormone

T&A   tonsillectomy and adenoidectomy

TAH   total abdominal hysterectomy; TAH and BSO if both ovaries removed as well

TIA   transient ischemic attack (a strokelike episode or neurologic symptom such as numbness or weakness that disappears completely within less than a day)

TIBC   total iron-binding capacity (measure of amount of blood proteins carrying iron)

tid   three times a day

TMJ   temporomandibular joint (the joint between the skull and the jawbone, a site of chronic pain or dysfunction)

TURP   transurethral resection of prostate (surgical chipping away of the prostate gland through the urethra to relieve blockage)

Tx, TX   treatment

UGI   upper GI series, barium X-ray of the esophagus, stomach, and duodenum

URI   upper respiratory infection

UTI   urinary tract infection

VS   vital signs

WBC   whole blood cell

WNL   within normal limits, normal findings

wt.   weight

X	times
x	except
↑	increase; high
↓	decrease; low
⚲ standing figure	standing
⚲ sitting figure	sitting
⚲ lying figure	lying
2°	secondary, due to or caused by

HOW TO WORK WITH THE HOSPITAL STAFF

Now that you know how to read the orders, you need to know how to ask questions without annoying anybody. The secret is to remember that this is not an us-against-them situation. The doctors, nurses, and aides are not the enemy. I'm always disturbed by advice from patients' rights activists that recommends an adversarial stance, as though you have to put up a fight to get your needs met. Maybe as an absolute last resort, when someone is clearly negligent, you'll have to get tough. But in general, as your mother probably told you, you'll catch more flies with honey than with vinegar. After all, most doctors and nurses went into a "helping profession" precisely because they want to help people. Give them the benefit of the doubt.

Let's say you ring the buzzer because the monitor connected to your mother's feeding tube is beeping. Minutes tick by with no response. When a nurse or an aide does finally show up, don't lash out and say "What took you so long?" Instead, glance at the person's name tag and then try something like this: "Oh, Mary, I'm so glad you're here. I was getting really nervous. What does that beeping sound mean anyway? Maybe I'm overreacting but I thought I'd better find out." Now you've got her on your side. You've addressed her by name and you've acknowledged that she has expertise which you don't have. She may be so flush with flattery that she'll give you a quick course in feeding tube technology. At the very least, Mary will check out the problem and leave with a good feeling about you.

She'll feel even better about you if you don't forget your manners. "Please" and "Thank you" are magic words when it comes to getting what you want. And, yes, it doesn't hurt to curry favor with an occasional gift. Like the schoolboy who brings an apple for the teacher and then gets chosen to be the line leader, you'll do well to butter up the staff by sharing that fruit basket or box of bonbons sent by a well-wisher. I speak from experience when I say that the nurses and aides will be grateful for the goodies. After all, they have to exist on cafeteria fare day in and day out!

Another tip: Get to know the staff and help them get to know you. Casual conversation while a nurse is fiddling with the IV or an aide is giving a sponge bath works wonders. Here's an example. You say, "Mary, you got a haircut! It looks great. Where did you have it done?" She smiles and tells you the name of the salon. You say, "That must be a new place. My mom always used to go to the one on Orchard Street when I was a little girl." Now your mother pipes up and says, "That was Diana's Beauty Shop. It's not there anymore. She retired." Suddenly your mother is not just another body to bathe, but a real person with some interesting history about the town. Your mother and Mary start talking and you chime in every now and then. The next time Mary comes in, she remembers your name and your mother's name and picks up the thread of the conversation. And when you let Mary know you're out of tissues, she's back with them in a flash.

HELP WITH DISCHARGE PLANNING AND GET YOUR DISCHARGE SUMMARY

There will probably be a team involved in the discharge—the hospitalist and/or family doctor, a nurse or two, and perhaps a social worker. Make certain you understand what the follow-up should be in terms of diet, exercise, medications, and return visits. Be certain that the team knows about any medications you (or the patient) had been taking before being admitted, and find out whether you should resume them and whether they might interact with new ones which have been prescribed.

When you're ready to leave the hospital, ask for a copy of the report which your attending doctor is required by law to dictate. Also, always ask for copies of your EKG and results of blood work and other tests if you are away from home and will need immediate follow-up care. The report won't be ready for a few weeks, so give the doctor a sticky note as a reminder and a self-addressed, stamped envelope. The summary will include why you came to the hospital, the results of your physical exams and laboratory tests, the differential diagnosis (list of possible causes of your problem) or assessment of your condition, treatment and procedures done while you were hospitalized, and the outcome, including whether you need further tests and medications and whether you need a follow-up. This comprehensive summary should automatically be sent to your family doctor if he was not the one who was in charge of your case. But as I have pointed out before, don't leave anything about your health care to chance. A friend of mine learned that getting the discharge summary later can be a lengthy and frustrating process. Janet's son was rushed to the emergency room with a combination of alcohol and acetaminophen poisoning after a night of partying with his college friends. His liver was severely damaged. However, the hospital in the college town did not send the report to Mike's doctor back home. Janet found that out because I'm in the habit of telling everyone I know to get copies of medical records. What follows is an e-mail I received from Janet chronicling her efforts to get the summary directly from the hospital:

"Hi!

Here's an update on trying to retrieve Mike's records from his stay at the university medical center back in February of 1999 with liver damage. I had Mike send a letter and a check to his primary doctor stating he would like copies of his medical file. The letter was dated Jan. 25, 2000. The doctor mailed out Mike's entire file Jan. 28, 2000. I should have had Mike be more specific! We got lots of papers with scribbling that I couldn't read. Anyway, I finally found a reference to the hospital stay, but it was not the discharge summary. Here's exactly what the primary doctor recorded: '2/16/99 412-123-4567 admitted U Med Center (Dr. John Doe) - tyl. overdose (accidental), showing liver damage has HealthAmerica - Dr. D ok'd - DR (178 32 3722)04- (HA will Review) 2-19-99 - still in hospital (AD) at U of Med Center.'

"There was no mention of the meds Mike was on or any treatment or whether he had any residual liver damage. I just figured the primary doctor followed through and would have a record of everything. NOT!

"Mike then sent a letter to the Med Center requesting his records. This was on Feb. 5, 2000. He got a letter back stating, 'need pt. auth or proof of next of kin.' Give me a break! I called and they said they had made an error and to resubmit the letter. Of course this was all a pain because Mike is in a dorm on campus and I'm at home and we had to keep calling back and forth. Mike sent another letter and this time he got a letter back stating, 'Your request for information regarding the above patient has been received. To further process this request, a prepayment of the reproduction fees for 63 pages is required. Please remit $68.28 to the address listed below and we will promptly process your request.' This was received on 4/30/2000. I checked the state law. The hospital is allowed to charge a dollar a page plus a handling fee. That's how they came up with the total fee. Again, we should have asked just for the summary, not for the whole file!

"I called the Med Center and they were nice and understanding and said they would charge only for the discharge summary. We finally got it. The scary part about this whole thing is if I didn't know you, I would have never thought to check on my Mike's records. If something ever happened to Mike that involved needing information about his liver damage, the result could have been a tragedy! From now on, I'm getting all our records as we go! Thanks for clueing me in!

Love ya,
Janet"

As Janet's story illustrates, reading your summary and giving a copy to your doctor and all subsequent doctors is critical. There is no one but you who will make absolutely sure that the right people have the information, especially if you are hospitalized while away from home. For example, if you have a hysterectomy, the pathology report from your surgery will show whether one or both ovaries were removed and/or your appendix. Believe it or not, many women aren't told this, and they don't ask.

Also, having all your summaries on hand when you need them is a big help in time of trouble. If you're diagnosed with cancer or a chronic condition, you may get a letter from a "new-patient coordinator" explaining that it is your responsibility to get all your records and discharge summaries together and send them to the oncologist or other specialist. Don't expect any sympathy. The tone of the letter is likely to be brisk and businesslike, leaving no doubt that you're just a number to the person who wrote it. One such letter from a leading hospital concludes with a less than comforting "There will be NO exceptions!" Wouldn't it be nice, if you ever did get such a letter, to be able to reach for your neat file of health records instead of going into panic mode when you're already overwhelmed with fear?

Enough said. You now know that the secret of getting good hospital care is to have a personal sentinel on hand who will chum with the staff and keep your spirits up at the same time. And you know that you have to arrange to have your discharge summary sent as soon as it's ready.

Now that you're on your way home, you no doubt have some instructions about what to do as you recuperate. Most of the directions, such as prudent diet and exercise regimens, are probably the good health habits you would have been wise to follow all along. Sometimes, a crisis such as a heart attack is enough to scare a person straight. Often, though, even high-risk patients find that making so-called lifestyle changes is very hard to accomplish. Statistics have long shown that a full 50 percent of patients don't do what the doctor ordered. In my view, that does not constitute a failure of patients to be "compliant" or "adherent," to use the buzz words of the hour. It represents a failure on the part of doctors to educate patients so that they have the knowledge, motivation, and techniques to follow through. When I speak to groups of doctors, I quote the following Chinese proverb: "Tell me and I will forget... Show me and I will remember... Involve me and I will understand."

Step 8, the culmination of my plan to help you save your own life, will involve you so that you will understand. You'll be able to take good care of yourself even if you've never been able to do that until now...

Step 8 Finding the Courage to Treat Yourself Right

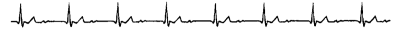

> *"Better to hunt in fields, for health unbought/*
> *Than fee the doctor for a nauseous draught/*
> *The wise, for cure, on exercise depend/*
> *God never made his work for man to mend."*
> —John Dryden

My dictionary defines the phrase "magic bullet" as follows: "1) A drug, therapy, or preventive therapy that cures or prevents a disease. 2) Something regarded as a magical solution to a grave problem or as a means of averting a disaster."

With the possible exception of antibiotics, modern medicine has no magic bullets. And even these "wonder drugs" are not meant to be used as substitutes for preventive measures such as simple hand washing, which can ward off infection in the first place. Insulin comes very close to qualifying as a magic bullet, but don't forget that people with Type 1 diabetes cannot manage the disease without careful attention to diet and exercise. Heart surgery doesn't count as an unqualified magic bullet either because an angioplasty or a bypass only correct harm already done and are no guarantee that the artery won't clog up again if the patient doesn't change his ways. Similarly, the new drugs which help counter the ravages of osteoporosis serve as an after-the-fact solution and won't work nearly as well if the patient doesn't stick to a regimen of balance and strength training and also improve her diet. Certainly, some diseases strike no

179

matter what you do, either because of heredity or plain bad luck. Even then, however, the better your health habits, the better your response will be to your treatment options. Ironically, Western doctors have not traditionally been trained in nutrition or exercise physiology. Yet simply put, no pill and no surgical procedure is ever a substitute for taking good care of yourself.

One patient who hated hearing that message was Barbara, the forty-nine-year-old woman we met in Step 6 when she was deciding whether or not to take hormone replacement therapy. A flamboyant person who liked rich food, strong drink, and unfiltered cigarettes, Barbara resisted the idea of giving up her indulgences. "You'd have to do a personality transplant on me if you wanted me to quit smoking, stop drinking, and start living on rabbit food," she said. "As for going to the gym, forget it! Maybe I'm killing myself, but I'm having a great time along the way. Anyway, it's probably too late now for damage control."

Lecturing Barbara was obviously not the way to go. But I had an ace up my sleeve. I knew that even though she *thought* she was "having a great time," she in fact didn't feel as well as she could. Barbara's behavior was not simply putting her at risk for such life-threatening diseases as lung cancer, diabetes, and heart disease. It was sapping her energy, dulling her taste buds, and saddling her with a chronic cough that left her with a sore throat and kept her from sleeping soundly. She also had frequent heartburn and suffered from aches and pains. Because she had gone on like this for so long, she didn't even realize how bad she felt. My plan was to get her to understand that, and then to agree to set a series of little goals. I was betting on the fact that once she started feeling better, she'd be inspired to keep cooperating so that a metamorphosis could occur—one that would not only be potentially life-saving, but would enhance the quality of her life and make it more worth living.

Maybe you're not as devil-may-care as Barbara was, and maybe the need to clean up your act isn't as great as hers was. Possibly you don't even have to be convinced that changes are in order. It could be that you have earnestly tried and yet failed more than once to lose weight or toss your cigarettes. Perhaps, like a lot of people, you've been beating up on yourself because you can't seem to quit smoking or stay on a healthy diet, and the idea that you're weak-willed has become a self-fulfilling prophecy. But whatever the case, the process through which I guided Barbara can help you, too. As she herself put it, "If I can reinvent myself, anybody can!"

RESETTING YOUR REMOTE CONTROL

We are creatures of habit. Once a behavior becomes ingrained, we perform it without even thinking. Try this little test. Move your telephone from one side of your desk or kitchen counter to the other. For the first few times the phone rings after that, even though your ears tell you where the sound is coming from, you'll automatically reach for the spot where the phone used to be. Here's another example. Let's say that everybody in your family always turns out the bathroom light before leaving. A houseguest comes to stay, and she leaves the light on. When you walk into the bathroom, even though your eyes see that the light is on, you will almost certainly reach for the light switch. Your brain is on automatic pilot, and it tells your arm to do what it usually does in that situation.

Obviously, relearning simple tasks is quick and easy. You'll be reaching for the phone in its new spot after only a couple of mistakes. Relearning complex behaviors such as changing your diet or quitting smoking is a lot more diffi-cult. But the principle is the same, and keeping that in mind is extremely helpful. For Barbara, reaching for a cigarette to go with her morning coffee had become a reflex action. Like a lot of smokers, she was so conditioned to light up that she was almost unaware of what she was doing. The same was true for her other risky habits. She was, as folk wisdom puts it, "set in her ways." But she wasn't *hopelessly* set in her ways. No one ever is. Understanding that fact is the key to believing that you can—with effort, desire, and support—*change* your ways.

DON'T TRY TO DO EVERYTHING AT ONCE

You're not going to die tomorrow morning if you don't revamp your entire lifestyle overnight. Barbara had to smile when I reminded her of that. "I'm not asking you to be superhuman," I said. "I'm not asking you to swear off the cigarettes, give up your martinis, pass up dessert, remember your medication, and start strength training all in one day. But if we don't begin somewhere, another year will slip by and you won't have reached any of your goals." Barbara nodded, still a little skeptical. "Let's make a phase-by-phase plan," I said. "I want you to start with something that is guar-anteed to have an intrinsic reward: regular exercise. If you do what I suggest, you'll breathe more easily, you'll sleep more soundly, your endorphins will kick in, your joints will be lubricated, and you'll probably get rid of those aches and pains." Barbara wrinkled up her nose, and said, "I *knew* you were going to make me join a gym!" I told her that I did hope she'd be doing some balance and strength training down the road so she could retain good posture and slow down the muscle loss that can come with age. But I reas-sured her that I wanted her to start with the easiest possible way to get moving. I suggested that she could park a little further from her destination, and not drive at all when she could reasonably walk instead.

Two weeks later, Barbara said she had done as I suggested and that she had to admit she was feeling peppier than she had in a long time. At that point, we made a reasonable timetable, putting Barbara's goals in order and giving her one or two months to work on each hoped-for achievement. She began to keep a journal, writing down how much she walked, exactly what she ate and drank, and how many cigarettes she smoked.

Barbara gained momentum and mental energy as she reached one goal after another. That is not to say, however, that she faced no obstacles. Here, for you to use, is what she learned along the way.

MAKE A HABIT OF IT

Like a lot of people, Barbara had trouble remembering to take her daily medication. She was on a mild diuretic to help lower her blood pressure, although our goal was to get her off the drug as her lifestyle changes began to do the job naturally. I also had Barbara take a multivitamin with 400 units of vitamin D to help her absorb calcium, and 400 units of folic acid to reduce the risk of heart disease and colon cancer. The supplement contained no iron because she was not menstruating any longer. Her other daily pills were calcium supplements, two at 600 milligrams each.

What helped Barbara remember the pills was to link them with her established morning ritual of brushing her teeth. She put the pills right out on the sink next to the toothpaste. She found that if she put the bottles in the medicine cabinet, she would overlook them.

Another tip: To remember to order refills, jot a note on your health calendar such as "One week supply of medication left. Call pharmacist" or "Prescription running out. Call doctor."

A CURE FOR THE COMMON SCOLD

A well-meaning spouse can turn into a nag when he's worried about your health. That's what happened to Barbara's husband. "He was never on my case before," she said. "But once he heard about the high blood pressure and all of my risks, he went ballistic. He was like, why are you still smoking? How can you eat that omelet when you know it's a heart attack on a plate? And on and on!" Barbara's solution: She clued Harry into her game plan and got him to cheer her on instead of bawl her out. She picked a calm moment when they were relaxing after dinner, and said, "I know you're worried about me, but please don't pressure me. The doc helped me work out a plan with little gradual increments. If I try to do everything at once, I'll totally backslide." Once she had let Harry in on her agenda, he eased up and started telling her he was proud of every step she took. And when she did slip a bit, he would reassure her that he believed in her and knew she could do better the next day.

THERE'S COMFORT IN NUMBERS

But when it came to support, Barbara didn't stop with Harry. "I'm about as tough a case as you could find," she said cheerfully. "I knew I needed all the help I could get." She was wise. Hearing coping strategies from people who are going through the same thing you are is a big help. Other patients are often the best teachers, and just knowing you're not alone is a relief. For Barbara, a circle of women friends who were all trying to eat right, exercise, and lose some weight served as an informal support group. One of the women had adult onset diabetes and she was rueful about not having lost weight before the disease caught up with her. That helped keep Barbara motivated.

To get herself to quit smoking, Barbara joined a health Web site with an interactive online "community" of quitters to give her tips and encouragement. And when Barbara got around to giving up drinking, she decided to join Alcoholics Anonymous. Anybody who drinks as much as Barbara did will probably need the tried-and-true twelve-step program offered by AA. Barbara fell into that category.

Note: Barbara was not dependent on any chemicals except alcohol and nicotine, but the group and step methods she used have been shown to be equally effective for people addicted to other substances. In some cases, inpatient rehabilitation is the best course of treatment.

SET THE DATE

For each of her goals, Barbara circled a date with special significance for her. You could do the same, picking a benchmark birthday or a wedding anniversary. Or you could give your child a "birthday present" by quitting smoking or starting an exercise program on his special day. Another idea is to join the millions of people who quit smoking every year in November as part of the American Cancer Society's annual "Great American Smokeout." Or be a part of the global village and quit in May during "World No Tobacco Day," sponsored by the World Health Organization, a program of the United Nations.

LIST WHAT'S HOLDING YOU BACK

Here is what Barbara wrote and how I responded to her:

1) This is like closing the barn door after the horse is out. I'm too far gone so why should I even try?

It's never too late. The human body is a miracle. Even when it's been mistreated for a long time, it will get busy with repair work if you give it a chance. For example, liver function will typically return to normal after you have quit drinking for only a few months.

2) How will I ever relax without a drink? When I'm stressed, booze is one thing that does it for me.

Alcohol is a central nervous system depressant. Your initial response may be an easing of stress, but in the long run—especially if you overdo—you're creating a vicious cycle in which you wake up vaguely out of sorts and start looking forward to alcohol to relieve the very symptoms it brought on. Stopping a dependence on alcohol is definitely not easy, but you'll actually feel less stressed if you do and sleep much better.

3) I'll never be able to concentrate without my cigarettes. I'm an accountant and unless I light up, I'm brain dead!

Some successful quitters use oral substitutes such as gum or hard candy to get past the withdrawal and keep their minds on their work. Other people find nicotine replacement therapy (NRT) useful. Nicotine is not harmful in itself. It's the carcinogens in smoke that are dangerous—both to you and the people around you. The NRT gums and patches deliver safe and gradually decreasing amounts of nicotine while you conquer your addiction. Some NRT products come with the offer of free support, including a hotline. Also, there is a smoking cessation drug available which was originally used for depression. You need a prescription. As you try to kick the habit, keep in mind that studies have shown that in one or two months after quitting smoking, the risk of dropping dead of a heart attack is significantly decreased. Also, the cilia— the "hairs" in the lungs—will "wake up" almost immediately and resume their job of cleaning out germs, which in turn will mean fewer respiratory infections. Better yet, within ten years of quitting smoking, your risk of lung cancer will be almost as low as if you had never smoked at all.

4) Food is my other comfort. I'll be a nervous wreck without my lasagna and my chocolate!

You don't have to sentence yourself to a lifetime of never touching your favorite foods again. Especially if you have a support group to keep you on track, you can work out ways to include some of what you love into your meal plan at least occasionally. However, you'll benefit from avoiding food binges. You can find new and healthy ways to relieve stress. Yoga works for many people and so does meditation. Courses are often offered at the local Y or at the high school as part of a continuing education program. Sign up with your health buddy so you'll both be motivated to go. And remember that as your weight goes down, so will your blood sugar and with it the risk of developing diabetes.

5) I hate taking meds. I look at a pill and I say to myself, great going, Barbara, you made yourself sick. I'd just rather not think about it.

Flip that around in your mind. Tell yourself you're glad that the pills are available to help you reach your goal. The medication is not, as I said, a magic bullet. But it can be an important part of the plan to reclaim your good health.

Your list will not necessarily be anything like Barbara's. Maybe you think you'll gain weight if you quit smoking. Or maybe your job requires a lot of restaurant meals with clients and you can't see how you'll ever stick to a healthy eating plan. Or perhaps you can't see how you could fit exercise into your already jammed schedule. Writing down each personal nemesis will make you face it squarely. Also, research has shown that writing about your health issues may be therapeutic in and of itself. Once you have identified your problems, get help from your doctor, health buddy, and your support group so you can begin to conquer them all.

SCARE YOURSELF

Barbara, who tended to live in the present and push away thoughts of what she might be doing to herself, resisted this idea at first. I decided to choose one of her trouble areas and lay out the ugly truth for her. "Smoking has been shown to cause cancer of the mouth, esophagus, and lung, not to mention wrinkling the skin," I said. "It can also cause emphysema, heart disease, and stroke. And secondhand smoke makes kids more prone to colds, ear infections, and allergies. It may stunt their growth and cause reading and behavior problems." Her eyes widened. "Now you've got me!" she said. "I've always been able to justify what smoking might be doing to my own body. But I've got a six-month-old granddaughter. You're telling me that if I smoke when I'm taking care of her, I'm making her sick and maybe screwing up her chances of doing well in school! Besides, now that you're forcing me to think about it, I know I want to stick around and see Callie grow up. Maybe I'd better get rid of my weeds after all."

For your part, talk with your doctor and use your research skills to learn what kind of jeopardy your current behavior is putting you in. Scare tactics can jump-start your willpower big time.

LAY IN SOME SUPPLIES

As you get ready to embark on a new health plan, stock up on items that can help you succeed, such as the following:

1) For quitting smoking, have a stash of bubble gum and lollipops and make sure you have something to do with your hands like knitting, crocheting, whittling, or crossword puzzles. Also, Barbara recommends buying NO SMOKING signs for your home, office, and car. She found this official act to be a great motivation.

2) To help yourself remember your medication, borrow Barbara's trick of keeping pills out where you can't help but see them. Also, get a portable pillbox with sections for the days of the week or for separate medications. Carry it with you in your purse or briefcase.

3) Buy a healthy-eating cookbook, and stock up on fresh fruits and vegetables, whole grains, fish and chicken, and fortified cottage cheese, plus herbs and spices.

4) If you can't or don't want to go to a gym, buy exercise videos and do your workout at home. You can choose a low-impact program if you have osteoporosis. And even if you're very limited in your ability to move, such as if you have rheumatoid arthritis, you can find "chair dancing" workouts that will do you a great deal of good.

GET RID OF REMINDERS OF YOUR OLD WAYS

1) If you're quitting smoking, have your carpets and clothes cleaned before your target date, and get your teeth cleaned as well.

2) Throw out ashtrays and cigarette holders.

3) If you're cutting down on alcohol or quitting altogether, put the martini shaker and the cocktail glasses away until company comes instead of leaving them where they're handy.

4) Toss out any leftover junk food.

WRITE A CONTRACT WITH YOURSELF

Put your goals on paper, spelling out exactly what you are promising yourself you will try to achieve. Sign and date the document. Get it out and read it when you feel your resolve weakening.

REWARD YOURSELF

On a regular basis—maybe once a week and at least once a month—give yourself a treat. Feeling good is a bonus in itself, as Barbara found out from the very beginning when she began her walking program. Still, an extra pat on the back every so often can't hurt. Some rewards can be inexpensive, such as going to a movie or playing hooky one afternoon to go to the beach. Others can be a little more pricey, especially if you're quitting smoking. Even if you only had a pack-a-day habit, you'll be saving over $1,000 a year. Spend some of it on whatever you like best—orchestra seats for the theater, a new set of golf clubs, or a mini-vacation at a luxury hotel. You earned it!

DO GOOD WHILE YOU'RE DOING WELL

Why not donate some of the money you used to spend on cigarettes, extra alcohol, and food to good causes such as the American Cancer Society or the American Heart Association? You might also want to become a peer counselor in a group such as Mended Hearts.

FOLLOW THE 1, 2, 3 OF PREVENTION FOR THE REST OF YOUR LIFE

There's an old joke that goes "I'd like some of that preventive medicine I keep hearing about." You now know that prevention is not a magic bullet but a way of life. Let's have a look at all the things you can do to stay as healthy as possible, using the three-stage model doctors are taught:

Primary prevention: This includes anything you do to keep a disease, condition, or injury from happening in the first place. The technical word is "prophylactic." Examples: wearing a helmet when you're riding a bike or skiing, buckling your seat belt in the car, getting all your shots when you need them, eating right, exercising regularly, de-stressing your life as much as possible, learning healthy ways to counter inevitable stress, staying on a regular sleep schedule, washing your hands frequently, avoiding putting your hands in your mouth and eyes, keeping rooms well ventilated, using humidifiers and dehumidifiers, practicing safe sex, using ergonomic chairs and keyboards, wearing sunglasses and goggles, wearing rubber gloves, using sunscreen, keeping a high hope outlook, and making sure you have a strong social support network of people who care about you.

Secondary prevention: This includes screening and diagnostic tests and procedures to detect health problems as early as possible, often before there are symptoms: blood tests to check for high cholesterol and myriad other conditions and diseases, blood pressure test to check for hypertension, EKG or cardiac stress test to rule out heart problems, Pap tests, colonoscopies, mammograms, and anything else you may need.

Tertiary prevention: This is rehabilitation—or as Barbara put it, damage control. Once you already have a disease or condition, it's still not too late to correct factors that contributed to it. Anything that helps you get better counts here, whether it's medication, surgery, physical therapy, diet, exercise, or quitting smoking. So that you can live well with your disease or condition, why not get ahold of the official guidelines for managing it? The information is intended for physicians and other health care professionals. However, as you know by now, I strongly believe you are capable of comprehending the material and that you deserve to know everything you can about how to take good care of yourself. You can find many guidelines on the Web (see Step 3, page 51), or you can ask your doctor for copies of the guidelines he uses. Also, you can write or call the organizations which publish guidelines. *Be sure to ask for the guidelines intended for professionals, not patients.*

American Academy of Allergy, Asthma, and Immunology: 414-272-6071

American Academy of Neurology, AAN Member Services Center (note: nonmembers can get the literature for a fee): 800-879-1960

American Academy of Pediatrics: 800-433-9016

American College of Cardiology, American Heart Association, Educational Services Department: 800-257-4740

American College of Obstetricians and Gynecologists: 800-762-2264

American College of Physicians: 800-523-1546

American College of Rheumatology: 404-633-3777

American Diabetes Association: 800-232-6733

American Medical Association: 312-464-5046

Federal Agency for Health Care and Policy Research: 800-358-9295

Step 8: Finding the Courage to Treat Yourself Right

National Heart, Lung and Blood Institute: NHLBI
Information Center, PO Box 30105, Bethesda, MD 20824-
0105; 301-251-1222

National Institute of Mental Health: 301-443-4513

National Institutes of Health: 888-644-2667

National Osteoporosis Foundation: 202-223-2226

US Preventive Services Task Force: 800-638-0672

Barbara did call for the official guidelines on managing hypertension and studied them herself. There is nothing like a convert! Halfway through the first year after her resolve to mend her ways, she had already dropped twenty pounds. She started urging all her friends to join her in her new life. "Who knew?" she said. "I had been dragging around with a hacking cough, creaky knees, and a perpetual hangover for years. And I thought that was the good life? No way! Now I'm a nut about this health stuff." Barbara says she is glad to know that she has lessened her chances of getting heart disease, diabetes, and osteoporosis. She's proud that she got to the point where she could control her high blood pressure without medication. And she's grateful that she looks and feels better than she ever thought she could.

But even though Barbara did a dramatic turnaround and took control of her health in so many ways, the specter of her inherited predisposition for breast cancer remained to haunt her. "After you told me that my family history puts me in the high-risk category, I started to obsess," she confided. "I lost my mom when I was only twenty years old. She never got to see her grandchildren. And I still miss her every single day. I used to be so damn flip about my health, but now that I'm on track, I want to live forever! I want to be there to see Callie graduate from high school, and then college, and then have a beautiful wedding that's over the top. I want to grow old with Harry. I know you keep telling me there's no magic bullet. But is there anything, anything at all I can do to help myself?"

I let a beat go by. The choices I could offer Barbara are far from perfect. But she deserved to know about them. "Remember what I told you about primary prevention?" I asked her. She nodded and said, "Sure, that's when you do something to keep from getting sick." Then I explained two options to prevent breast cancer. First, I told her about a preventive medication, but I let her know that it carries with it a lot of risks including increased risk of uterine cancer and blood clots, and that it is only recommended for five years. "That's a lousy crap shoot!" Barbara shot back. "What's the other option?" I then explained the double prophylactic mastectomy. "Critics say it's unnecessary mutilation," I said. "But the statistics for a woman as high-risk as you happen to be are worth looking at. A full 85 percent to 90 percent of women who have the procedure don't get breast cancer." Barbara was very quiet for a long while. "So I get them both cut off, but then chances are that I'll live to have my golden years with Harry, and I get to see Callie grow up. Listen, I've always been a gambler at heart. I like the odds here. Where do I sign up?" I then mentioned that genetic counseling might help her make a fully informed decision. This is a history taken by a trained counselor. Tests may be involved but they are not foolproof. Also, even if a woman doesn't have the gene, a family history like Barbara's can strongly predispose her to breast cancer. Barbara took a couple of weeks to think about all of this and talk things over with Harry. Then she called me and said she didn't want to have the genetic counseling but that she did want to have the prophylactic surgery.

If there were ever an example of having the courage to

treat yourself right, Barbara's brave decision is it. You may not agree with her. But that's not the point. We are individuals. With all the facts in front of us, we need to weigh the pros and cons and make what we believe are the right choices as we put forth every effort to save our own lives. Whether you are simply learning to change your eating habits or whether you are making a decision as bold as the one Barbara made, you are the one in charge. And that makes all the difference. Remember, prevention and long-term disease management are not really your doctor's job. They're yours. Once you're in control and doing all you can do, you have the greatest chance of not getting sick in the first place—and of getting better or at least feeling as well as possible if you do.

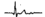

By now, you know that I have a genuine sense of mission about spreading my message. The epilogue of this book sums up the reasons I feel so strongly that my eight steps will always be essential, no matter what the future of health care may hold. I think you'll agree . . .

Epilogue

Here's to Your Health!

"Health is the greatest of human blessings."
—Hippocrates

I can't do anything to make your insurance plan less complicated. I can't keep your employer from switching plans and forcing you to change doctors. I can't keep HMOs from going bankrupt, leaving you to scramble for another insurer. I can't increase the number of nurses on hospital staffs. I can't snap my fingers and bring into being a secure nationwide system of computerized medical records and "smart cards."

What I can do is encourage you to make the best of a bad situation. As I see it, pointing the finger of blame is a colossal waste of time. The insurance companies might seem to be an easy target. But remember that while you may not like the fact that your plan asks your doctor to justify every test he orders or puts a limit on how much physical therapy you can have, it is the insurance companies' emphasis on prevention—theoretically resulting in fewer sick people filing claims—that has prompted them to cover tests and procedures such as the Pap smear and the sigmoidoscopy. Many plans also encourage a healthy lifestyle by providing educational materials about diet, exercise, fitness, and quitting smoking.

What about the doctors? They've been accused of having blinders on, focusing on their own practices while the insurance companies took the reins and rendered physicians less able to give their patients adequate time and attention. Maybe so. But bemoaning that fact won't change it, any more than complaining about the insurance companies will. Also, waiting around for computerized records, which have been promised since the 1970s at least, isn't going to give you the control you need right this minute over your own health care.

Anyway, even if we did have "smart cards" and computerized medical records, they wouldn't erase the need for following my eight steps. Nothing will ever replace trusting your intuition, keeping providers abreast of all your health information, being well informed yourself, getting shots and tests when you need them, establishing an interactive rapport with your doctor instead of cowering in his presence, taking part in decisions about your treatment, teaming up with a health buddy especially when you go to the hospital, and safeguarding your health by living right. What this all boils down to is taking charge of your medical care. Interestingly, that in itself translates into a major health benefit. Research shows that when you are not in control of a situation, your immune system may be compromised. Yet when you cease to feel helpless, even if you have a chronic or life-threatening condition, your immune system kicks back in—and so does your will to do all you can to prevent, fight, and manage disease and disability.

You really do have the power to save your own life. It's never too early and never too late to begin. Start now, and take it one step at a time. You'll be very glad you did.

Appendix

Copies of Actual Medical Records

Complete Male Blood Test

SB SmithKline Beecham — Clinical Laboratories

LABORATORY REPORT

Patient Name	Patient ID/Hospital ID	Room No	Age	Sex	Physician
			50	M	FENTON, BRADLEY

Page	Requisition No.	Accession No.	Lab Ref No.	Collection Date & Time	Log-in Date	Report Date & Time
1	0001547	KP430082L	0001547	12/01/98 10:39	12/01/98	12/03/98 06:00

Remarks

SS#: 174-30-8458

Report Status	Test	Result In Range	Out of Range	Units	Reference Range	Site Code
FINAL						
	LIPID PANEL					
	TRIGLYCERIDES	135		MG/DL	<200	KP
	CHOLESTEROL, TOTAL	186		MG/DL	<200	KP
	HDL-CHOLESTEROL	53		MG/DL	> 34	KP
	%8841SB* LDL-CHOLESTEROL	106		MG/DL (CALC)	0-130	KP
	%8842SB* CHOL/HDLC RATIO	3.51		(CALC)	<4.98	KP
	COMPREHENSIVE METABOLIC PANEL					
	GLUCOSE	90		MG/DL	70-125	KP
	UREA NITROGEN (BUN)	16		MG/DL	7-25	

Test	Value	Flag	Units	Reference Range	
SODIUM	1̶3̶1̶		MEQ/L		
POTASSIUM	4.3		MEQ/L	3.5-5.3	
CHLORIDE	102		MEQ/L	95-108	
CALCIUM	9.6		MG/DL	8.5-10.3	
PROTEIN, TOTAL	7.4		G/DL	6.0-8.5	
ALBUMIN	4.2		G/DL	3.2-5.0	
GLOBULIN	3.2		G/DL (CALC)	2.2-4.2	
ALBUMIN/GLOBULIN RATIO	1.3		(CALC)	0.8-2.0	
BILIRUBIN, TOTAL	0.7		MG/DL	0.0-1.3	
ALKALINE PHOSPHATASE	40		U/L	20-125	
AST (SGOT)	26		U/L	0-42	KP

CBC (INCLUDES DIFF/PLT)

Test	Value	Flag	Units	Reference Range	
WHITE BLOOD CELL COUNT	4.0		THOUS/MCL	3.8-10.8	
RED BLOOD CELL COUNT	4.53		MILL/MCL	4.40-5.80	
HEMOGLOBIN	14.1		G/DL	13.8-17.2	
HEMATOCRIT		40.4 L	%	41.0-50.0	
MCV	89.2		FL	80.0-100.0	
MCH	31.1		PG	27.0-33.0	
MCHC	34.9		%	32.0-36.0	
RDW	13.9		%	9.0-15.0	
PLATELET COUNT	208		THOUS/MCL	130-400	
ABSOLUTE NEUTROPHILS	2640		CELLS/MCL	1500-7800	
NEUTROPHILS	66		%		
ABSOLUTE LYMPHOCYTES	960		CELLS/MCL	850-4100	
LYMPHOCYTES	24		%		
ABSOLUTE MONOCYTES	360		CELLS/MCL	200-1100	
MONOCYTES	9		%		
ABSOLUTE EOSINOPHILS		40 L	CELLS/MCL	50-550	
EOSINOPHILS	1		%		
ABSOLUTE BASOPHILS	0		CELLS/MCL	0-200	
BASOPHILS	0		%		KP

URINALYSIS, REFLEX
| COLOR | YELLOW | | | YELLOW | KP |

>> REPORT CONTINUED ON NEXT PAGE <<

continued on next page

Complete Male Blood Test continued

SB *SmithKline Beecham*
Clinical Laboratories

LABORATORY REPORT

Patient Name		Patient ID/Hospital ID		Room No.	Age	Sex	Physician
					60	M	FENTON, BRADLEY

Page	Requisition No.	Accession No.	Lab Ref No.		Collection Date & Time	Log-in Date	Report Date & Time
2	0001547	KP4300082L	0001547		12/01/98 10:39	12/01/98	12/03/98 06:00

Remarks

SS#: 174-30-8458

Report Status	FINAL	Test	Result in Range / Out of Range	Units	Reference Range	Site Code
URINALYSIS, REFLEX (CONTINUED)						
	APPEARANCE		CLEAR		CLEAR	
	SPECIFIC GRAVITY		1.012		1.001-1.035	
	PH		6.5		4.6-8.0	
	GLUCOSE		NEGATIVE		NEGATIVE	
	BILIRUBIN		NEGATIVE		NEGATIVE	
	KETONES		NEGATIVE		NEGATIVE	
	OCCULT BLOOD		NEGATIVE		NEGATIVE	
	PROTEIN		NEGATIVE		NEGATIVE	
	NITRITE		NEGATIVE		NEGATIVE	
	LEUKOCYTE ESTERASE		NEGATIVE		NEGATIVE	
PROSTATE SPECIFIC ANTIGEN (HYBRITECH)						KP

Return to site: SOUTH...........
400 EGYPT ROAD
NORRISTOWN PA 19403
(215) 631-4200

>> END OF REPORT <<

Typical Female Blood Test

PATIENT

REQ: D9332488-0

COL. TIME: 2:30 PM

ACCESSION NO. 5494051-2

REQUESTED BY
SAVARD, MARIE
191 PRESIDENTIAL BLVD./44
BALA CYNWYD, PA 19004

AGE	SEX	COLLECTION DATE	ACCESSION DATE	REPORT DATE	ACCOUNT NO.	FRAME	ROUTE
NI	F	02/01/93	02/02/93	02/03/93	22053	132300645	967

TEST NAME	PATIENT'S RESULTS WITHIN RANGE	OUTSIDE RANGE	REFERENCE RANGE	UNITS
TESTS ORDERED: SED RATE, WINTROBE, F-ANA, CBC, CHEM, CANCER ANTIGEN 125, THYROID GROUP 6000.				
BLOOD COUNTS:				
WBC COUNT	6.3		4.0-11.0	THOUS/MM3
RBC COUNT	4.51		M:4.4-6.2 F:3.8-5.4	MILL/MM3
HEMOGLOBIN	13.6		M:13-18 F:11.5-16	GM/DL
HEMATOCRIT	39.1		M:39-54 F:35-48	%
MCV	87		80-100	FL
MCH	30.1		27.0-33.0	PG
MCHC	34.7		31.0-36.0	%
SEGS	55		40-74	%
LYMPHS	34		19-48	%
MONOS	9		0-13	%
EOSINS	1		0-7	%
BASOS	1		0-3	%
PLATELETS	294		130-400	THOUS/MM3

WINTROBE ESR	4		M:0-9 F:0-20	MM/HR
BLOOD CHEMISTRY, ROUTINE:				
GLUCOSE, SERUM	89		65-115	MG/DL
BUN	19		7-25	MG/DL
CREATININE	1.0		0.6-1.5	MG/DL
BUN/CREAT RATIO	19.0		9.0-24.0	RATIO
SODIUM	146		135-147	MEQ/L
POTASSIUM	4.2		3.5-5.3	MEQ/L
CHLORIDE	107		96-109	MEQ/L
URIC ACID	2.9		M:3.0-9.0 F:2.2-7.7	MG/DL
T.PROTEIN	6.6		6.0-8.5	GM/DL
ALBUMIN	4.3		3.5-5.5	GM/DL
GLOBULIN	2.3		2.0-3.5	GM/DL
A/G RATIO	1.9		1.0-2.4	RATIO
CALCIUM	9.2		8.5-10.8	MG/DL
PHOSPHATE	3.6		2.5-4.5	MG/DL
ALK PHOS	35		ADULT:25-140	U/L
SGOT (AST)	18		0-40	U/L
SGPT (ALT)	9		0-45	U/L
LDH	121		100-225	U/L
BILIRUBIN, TOTAL	0.5		0.0-1.2	MG/DL
BILIRUBIN, DIRECT	0.2		0.0-0.5	MG/DL
GAMMA-GTP	11		M:9-65 F:7-37	U/L

Thomas J. Liddy M.D.

THOMAS J. LIDDY, M.D.
LABORATORY DIRECTOR

NOTE: Stated ranges and flagging of results represent only
nominal normal values. Interpretation of test results should
be considered in the light of patient age and sex together
with any medications the patient is using. See also important information on reverse side.

continued on next page

Typical Female Blood Test continued

PATIENT:

REQ: D9332488-0   TIME: 2:30 PM

| ACCESSION NO. | 5494051-2 |

REQUESTED BY

SAVARD, MARIE
191 PRESIDENTIAL BLVD. /44
BALA CYNWYD, PA 19004

AGE	SEX	COLLECTION DATE	ACCESSION DATE	REPORT DATE	ACCOUNT NO.	PRIME	ROUTE
NI	F	02/01/93	02/02/93	02/03/93	22053	132300645	967

TEST NAME	PATIENT'S RESULTS WITHIN RANGE	PATIENT'S RESULTS OUTSIDE RANGE	REFERENCE RANGE	UNITS
FERRITIN	88		SEE BELOW	NG/ML
MALES: 20-450 FEMALES: <45 YRS: 8-200; >45 YRS: 10-350				
BLOOD LIPIDS/CHD RISK ASSESSMENT:				
TOTAL CHOLESTEROL		234 HI	130-200	MG/DL
TRIGLYCERIDES	42		30-150	MG/DL
HDL CHOLESTEROL		79	M:30-75 F:40-90	MG/DL
LDL CHOLESTEROL, CAL		147 HI	<130 DESIRABLE	MG/DL
CHOL/HDL RATIO	3.0		SEE BELOW	RATIO

	MALE	FEMALE
LOWEST CHD RISK	<3.5	<3.5
BELOW AVERAGE CHD RISK	3.5-4.4	3.5-4.4

	DANGEROUS	CHD RISK	>13.4	>10.9	

THYROID EVALUATION:

T3 UPTAKE RATIO	1.02		0.80-1.20	RATIO
T4 (RIA)	10.4		4.5 - 12.5	MCG/DL
FREE T4 INDEX	10.6		4.0-12.3	INDEX
T-3 (RIA)	116		80-220	NG/DL
TSH	1.6		0.4-6.0	uIU/ML

IMMUNOLOGY, ROUTINE:

FANA	NEGATIVE		NEGATIVE <1:40	TITER

CANCER ANTIGEN 125:

CA-125, SERUM	14		LESS THAN 35	U/ML

CA-125 IS ELEVATED IN APPROXIMATELY 1% OF HEALTHY
INDIVIDUALS AND MAY BE ELEVATED IN PREGNANCY AND
OTHER BENIGN AND MALIGNANT DISEASES. A CA-125
VALUE LESS THAN 35 U/ML DOES NOT INDICATE ABSENCE
OF RESIDUAL OVARIAN CANCER.

*** F I N A L ***

Thomas J. Liddy MD

THOMAS J. LIDDY, M.D.
LABORATORY DIRECTOR

NOTE: Stated ranges and flagging of results represent only
nominal normal values. Interpretation of test results should
be considered in the light of patient age and sex together
with any medications the patient is using. See also important information on reverse side.

Generic Blood Test, Male or Female

Patient Name		Patient ID	Age	Sex	Date Collected	Time Collected		Accession No.
MARIE S			44	F	10/09/97	02:00		109314372
	Requesting Physician/Remarks				Date Received	Date Reported	Report Status	Page
					10/10/97	10/11/97	FINAL	1

Test	Out of Range	Results — Within Range	Reference Range	Units
CS 24, HDL				
CS 24 (22 CHEM)				
CALCIUM, SERUM		8.9	8.4-10.2	MG/DL
PHOSPHORUS, SERUM		3.3	2.3-4.6	MG/DL
MAGNESIUM, SERUM		1.9	1.8-2.6	MG/DL
GLUCOSE	132 H		65-114	MG/DL
BUN		16	7-23	MG/DL
CREATININE, SERUM		0.8	0.6-1.5	MG/DL
BUN CREATININE RATIO		20	7-24	
URIC ACID, SERUM		3.5	2.2-6.8	MG/DL
CHOLESTEROL		192	<200	MG/DL
TRIGLYCERIDE		73	<200	MG/DL
TOTAL PROTEIN, SERUM		6.9	6.0-8.2	G/DL
ALBUMIN		4.6	3.5-5.0	G/DL
GLOBULIN		2.3	1.9-3.8	G/DL
A-G RATIO		2.0	0.9-2.1	G/DL
BILIRUBIN, TOTAL		0.8	0.2-1.4	MG/DL
BILIRUBIN, DIRECT		0.3	0.0-0.4	MG/DL

Test		Value	Reference Range	Units
AST/SGOT		32	1-40	U/L
ALT/SGPT		34	1-50	U/L
LDH		128	110-250	U/L
SODIUM, SERUM		140	134-145	MEQ/L
POTASSIUM, SERUM		3.6	3.5-5.3	MEQ/L
CHLORIDE, SERUM		98	96-107	MEQ/L
IRON, TOTAL SERUM	200 H		29-162	MCG/DL
HDL		76	30-85	MG/DL
CHOL/HDL RATIO		2.5	SEE REVERSE	
LDL (CALCULATED)		101	<160	MG/DL
LDL/HDL RATIO		1.3	SEE REVERSE	
CBC (INCLUDES DIFF AND PLATELET)				
WBC		8.1	3.9-11.4	THOUS/UL
RBC		4.29	3.80-5.10	MIL/UL
HEMOGLOBIN		14.0	11.6-15.2	G/DL
HEMATOCRIT		40.4	34.0-45.0	%

PAGE 1: CONTINUED ON PAGE 2

Herman Hurwitz, M.D., F.C.A.P., Senior Medical Director • Robert M. Lucas, M.D., D.D.S., Ph.D., Associate Medical Director • Maryam Bakhtar, M.D., F.C.A.P., Anatomic Pathology, Director
Vivian Anagnoste, M.D., Pathologist • Jose Reyes, M.D., Pathologist • Katherine Erickson, Ph.D., Technical Director

continued on next page

Generic Blood Test, Male or Female continued

Patient Name	Patient ID	Age	Sex	Date Collected	Time Collected	Accession No.
MARIE S		44	F	10/09/97	02:00	109314392
Requesting Physician / Remarks				Date Received	Date Reported	Report Status
				10/10/97	10/11/97	FINAL Page 3

Test	Results Out of Range	Within Range	Reference Range	Units
ANA FLUORESCENT		< 1:40	< 1:40	
RHEUMATOID FACTOR, SERUM		< 1:20	< 1:20	
	* END OF FINAL REPORT *			
	Printed on: 10/11/97 at: 10:53 AM			

Upon completion of laboratory studies, a duplicate report will
be forwarded to the consulting physician per your request.

Duplicate report to: DR. FRANK MARCHLINSKI

Typical Chest X-ray

Graduate Plaza
1438397--PDP
Copy 1

THE GRADUATE HOSPITAL
DIAGNOSTIC RADIOLOGY/NUCLEAR MEDICINE

M. BROOKS, M.D.
A. CHAIT, M.D.

W.S. CYNN, M.D.
J.G. JACOBSTEIN, M.D.

F. KRAMER, M.D.
B.L. LEVIN, M.D.

D.P. MAYER, M.D.
M. MURDOCK, M.D.

J.D. RUBIN, M.D.
L.P. SIMERMAN, M.D.

ACCOUNT NO.

LAST NAME 740504   DATE OF EXAMINATION 06/12/92

FIRST NAME/M.I.

Marie Savard, M.D.
191 Presidential Blvd.
Bala Cynwyd, PA 19004

DOB: 09/21/53
female

AGE 38Y   PROCEDURE /Chest/   (CB)   Outpatient

RTED BY   Jon Cynn, M.D.

approved by WC on 06/16/92

REPORT

CHEST - CODE 71020

IMPRESSION:
NO ACTIVE PROCESS.

COMMENT:
PA AND LATERAL VIEWS OF THE CHEST WERE EVALUATED WITHOUT
PRIOR STUDIES FOR COMPARISON. THE LUNGS ARE WELL EXPANDED AND
THERE MAY BE SMALL SCATTERED GRANULOMAS. THERE IS NO ACTIVE
INFILTRATION. THERE IS A SMALL NODULAR DENSITY OVER THE RIGHT
LOWER LUNG, MOST LIKELY REPRESENTING NIPPLE SHADOW. THE
CARDIOVASCULAR SILHOUETTE IS WITHIN NORMAL LIMITS.

CB

Bone Density—Early Osteoporosis

PATIENT ID:
NAME:

SCAN: 1.31 04/01/97
ANALYSIS: 1.31 04/01/97

ID: SCAN DATE: 04/01/97

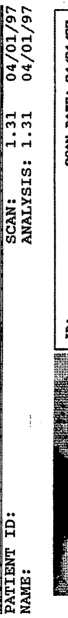

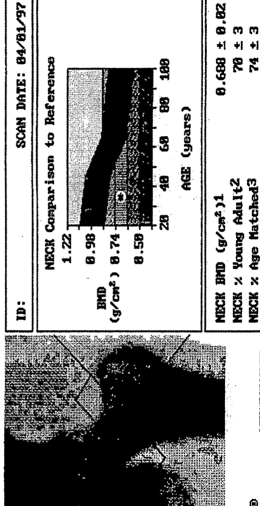

NECK Comparison to Reference

BMD (g/cm^2)	
1.22	
0.98	
0.74	
0.50	

AGE (years): 20   40   60   80   100

NECK BMD (g/cm^2)1   0.688 ± 0.02
NECK % Young Adult2   70 ± 3
NECK % Age Matched3   74 ± 3

LUNAR®

Weight (lb)..........	114.0	Small Standard......	140.72
Height (in)..........	67	Low keV Air (cps)...	791399
Ethnic...............	White	High keV Air (cps)..	466222
System...............	7718	Rvalue (%Fat).......	1.385(5.1)
Side.................	Left	Current (uA)........	3000

Collimation (mm).....	1.68
Sample Size (mm).....	1.2x 1.2
Region height (mm)...	60.0
Region width (mm)....	15.0
Region angle (deg)...	51

NECK	:	BMC^5 (grams) =	3.22	$AREA^5$ (cm^2) =	4.68
WARDS	:	BMC^5 (grams) =	1.53	$AREA^5$ (cm^2) =	2.43
TROCH	:	BMC^5 (grams) =	4.98	$AREA^5$ (cm^2) =	8.50

REGION	BMD^1 g/cm^2	Young Adult[2] %	Z	Age Matched[3] %	Z
NECK	0.688	70	-2.43	74	-2.02
WARDS	0.631	69	-2.14	74	-1.69
TROCH	0.586	74	-1.85	78	-1.49

1 - See appendix E on precision and accuracy. Statistically 68% of repeat scans will fall within 1 SD.

2 - USA Femur Reference Population, Ages 20-45. See Appendices.

3 - Matched for Age, Weight(males 25-100kg; females 25-100kg), Ethnic.

5 - Results for research purposes, not clinical use.

Bone Density—Severe Osteoporosis

PATIENT ID:
NAME:

SCAN: 1.31 04/01/97
ANALYSIS: 1.31 04/01/97

ID: SCAN DATE: 04/01/97

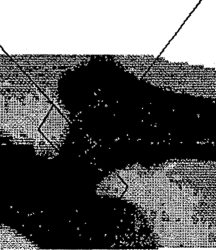

NECK Comparison to Reference

BMD (g/cm^2)

1.22	
0.98	
0.74	
0.50	

AGE (years)
20 40 60 80 100

NECK BMD (g/cm^2)1   0.725 ± 0.02
NECK % Young Adult2   74 ± 3
NECK % Age Matched3   93 ± 3

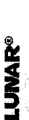

LUNAR®

Height (in)......... 66   Collimation (mm)...... 1.68

Ethnic.............. White   Sample Size (mm)...... 1.2x 1.2

System.............. 7718   Region height (mm).... 60.0

Side................ Left   Region width (mm)..... 15.0

   (...) Standard...... 140.72   Region angle (deg)... 50

Low keV Air (cps)... 791399

High keV Air (cps).. 466222

Rvalue (%Fat)....... 1.345(23.7)

Current (uA)........ 3000

NECK   : BMC^5 (grams) = 3.36 $AREA^5$ (cm^2) = 4.64
WARDS   : BMC^5 (grams) = 1.41 $AREA^5$ (cm^2) = 2.39
TROCH   : BMC^5 (grams) = 7.41 $AREA^5$ (cm^2) = 12.66

REGION	BMD^1 g/cm^2	Young Adult[2] %	Young Adult[2] Z	Age Matched[3] %	Age Matched[3] Z
NECK	0.725	74	-2.13	93	-0.47
WARDS	0.587	65	-2.48	92	-0.41
TROCH	0.585	74	-1.86	86	-0.88

1 - See appendix E on precision and accuracy. Statistically 68% of repeat scans will fall within 1 SD.

2 - USA Femur Reference Population, Ages 20-45. See Appendices.

3 - Matched for Age, Weight(males 25-100kg; females 25-100kg), Ethnic.

5 - Results for research purposes, not clinical use.

CT of Abdomen

OUTPATIENT   F25 (08/15/

02/10/99 CT ABD/PELVIS W/CON

ORDERED BY: Dr. Adam C. Sobel

DIAGNOSIS:

Normal CT examination of the abdomen.

COMMENT:

A CT examination of the abdomen was performed with IV and oral contrast.   There are no prior studies for comparison.

Clinical history given is: Abdominal pain and left side rib pain.

Examination of the abdomen is unremarkable.   The liver, spleen, pancreas, adrenals, kidneys, and gallbladder are normal.   The lung bases are clear.   Evaluation of the bony structures demonstrates no lytic or blastic lesions.

This exam and the report were personally reviewed by Dr. Wechsler, who agrees with the findings.

Dictated and signed: Richard J. Wechsler, M.D./Douglas Montgomery, M.D.
Mailed: 02/17/99 7:36 am

Mammogram

January 24, 1994

Marie Savard, M.D.
191 Presidential Blvd.
Suite W-1
Bala Cynwyd, PA 19004

RE:

Comparison Study

Dear Dr. Savard:

Thank you for the opportunity of examining your patient,
on January 24, 1994.

An examination from Metropolitan Hospital dated 1/8/90 is now
available for comparison with our recent examination. When
comparison is made, no changes are noted. No new dominant masses,
spiculations, or clustered microcalcifications are seen to suggest
malignancy. Continued annual mammographic follow-up is
recommended.

Impression: No change in comparison with the previous outside
radiographs.

Sincerely,

C. Amy Wilson, M.D.

CAW/lt

EKG

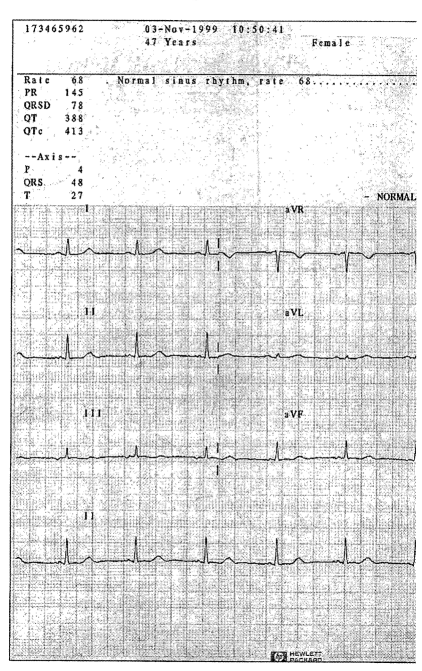

Normal P axis, PR, rate & rhythm

Requested by:
FENTON

Unconfirmed diagnosis.

V1   V4

V2   V5

V3   V6

25 mm/s   10 mm/mV   ∿ 0.15 Hz - 40 Hz   HP708   01570
REORDER HP M2481A.

Cardiac ECHO

Name   Date <u>August 6, 1992</u>   Age 43   Sex M

Hospital   Room # C-350   File # 288-92   Tape # 92-130

        HT.   WT.   Referring   R.P.

Referral Codes: Effusion Valve fct.

FINDINGS:

1. <u>M-MODE AND TWO-DIMENSIONAL ECHO INTERPRETATION</u>

A mechanical prosthesis is noted in the aortic position. The left
atrium is at the upper limits of normal in size. There is the
appearance of mild mitral valve prolapse. The mitral leaflets open
normally during diastole. The left ventricle is normal in size
with excellent contractility. There is mild abnormal septal
motion. There is mild concentric left ventricular hypertrophy. No
pericardial effusion is seen. The right sided cardiac structures
appear normal.

2. DOPPLER OBSERVATIONS

This is consistent with mild mitral regurgitation as well as mild
tricuspid regurgitation. There was pulmonic insufficiency noted.
No aortic insufficiency was seen. Continuous wave Doppler across
the aortic prosthesis fail to suggest obstruction of the
prosthesis.

CONCLUSIONS:

1. No pericardial effusion.
2. Good left ventricular contractility with borderline left
   ventricular hypertrophy.
3. Borderline enlargement of the left atrium.
4. Mild regurgitant lesions as noted above.
5. Abnormal septal motion consistent with the post surgical state.

Gary J. Vigilante, M.D.
Co-Director
Cardiac Ultrasound Laboratory

Medical Center is an affiliate of the University of Pennsylvania

```
Name                    Date August 6, 1992    Age 43    Sex M

Hospital # 52-98-94    Room # C-350  File # 288-92  Tape # 92-130

DOB 6-1-49   HT.    WT.   Referring Silber   Tech R.P.


                    QUANTITATIVE MEASUREMENTS

Chamber Dimensions

Aortic Root                      36 mm          (20-37mm)

LA                               53 mm          (19-40mm)

RV(diastole)                     28 mm          ( 5-25mm)

LV(diastole)                     55 mm          (23-56mm)

LV(systole)                      26 mm

LV wall thickness

Septum                           12 mm          (7-11mm)

Post. wall                       13 mm          (7-11mm)

LV mass

Valve Measurements

Aortic leaflet opening           AVR mm          (16-26mm)

Mitral leaflet E-F slope         105 mm/sec    (80-150 mm/sec)

Mitral valve D-E Excursion       20 mm          (20-30 mm)

Mitral E-point-septal separation 3 mm          (< 7 mm)

Hemodynamics

Ejection Fraction                %              (< 55%)

Cardiac output                   l/m


Pericardium

Effusion                         mm

Thickness                        mm
```

Typical Typed Consultation

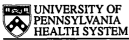
March 13, 1997

Marie Savard Fenton, M.D.
191 Presidential Boulevard
Suite W-1
Bala Cynwyd, PA 19004

Re:
NRN:

Dear Dr. Savard:

On January 31, 1997 I had the pleasure of evaluating   for a second opinion regarding her persistent complaints of intermittent shortness of breath. I would have to say in brief that my conclusions were essentially those of Sweinberg from her initial evaluation of ⌐ on February 27, 1996. In essence I feel that Mrs.   as reactive airways disease possibly induced by her previous smoking history as well as her multiple episodes of upper respiratory tract infections manifested predominantly by tracheobronchitis. In addition, she has persistent and active chronic rhinitis and sinusitis which is probably a significant contributor as well. The presence of birds and two dogs in her home may also be a significant problem.

Her physical examination was most significant for the presence of very inflamed edematous nasal turbinates bilaterally and a question of cobblestoning over the posterior pharynx. Her pulmonary examination showed excellent air movement bilaterally with no evidence of wheezes or rhonchi and quiet expiration, but she did have fairly diffuse expiratory wheezes on forced expiratory maneuvers. Review of her x-rays and CT scans revealed a stable benign-appearing left lower lobe solitary pulmonary nodule which has been unchanged since April of 1996.

It was my impression as it was Dr. Sweinberg's that the patient may well benefit from an inhaled nasal corticosteroid to decrease her symptoms of chronic rhinitis, sinusitis, and possibly her reactive airways disease. I felt that she would also benefit from continued prn use of her beta agonists for her episodic shortness of breath. She may also benefit from removing her pets from her home if she has not already done so.

One of the patient's concerns was whether she had "early emphysema." Based upon her previous pulmonary function tests performed one year ago there was no evidence that this was an occurrence, but I have told her that to rule this out we would need to obtain full pulmonary function tests with lung volumes and a diffusion capacity. If these demonstrated a significant abnormality we might consider sending an alpha-1 antitrypsin level to rule out any genetic predisposition for the development of early emphysema. I also told her that the likelihood of either of these things being abnormal was quite low.

I apologize for the delay in getting this letter to you, but I want to thank you for your referral of this very pleasant woman for evaluation at the University of Pennsylvania Medical Center Pulmonary and Critical Care Program.

Should you have any specific questions regarding her evaluation, please feel free to contact me at any time.

Sincerely yours,

Daniel H. Sterman, M.D.
University of Pennsylvania Medical Center

DHS:jmb

223

Typical Typed Consultation

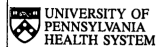 UNIVERSITY OF
PENNSYLVANIA
HEALTH SYSTEM

Department of Otorhinolaryngology:
Head and Neck Surgery

December 26, 1997

Marie Savard-Fenton, M.D.
191 Presidential Boulevard
Suite W1
Bala Cynwyd, PA 19004

RE:

Dear Dr. Savard-Fenton:

I had the pleasure of seeing   follow-up today. She notes that she has had three ear infections in the right ear since June and was last treated about two weeks ago. She feels as if the hearing has decreased some and she has lost the hearing aid for her left ear.

On examination she was very pleasant, alert, and in no acute distress. She had very narrow ear canals bilaterally which were obstructed by cerumen. This was debrided. The tympanic membranes were intact and the middle ears were clear bilaterally. She does have some scarring in the right ear secondary to her previous surgery. The remainder of her head and neck examination was unremarkable. We will get her set-up for a repeat audiometric evaluation as she does have some underlying hearing loss and she will also see the audiologist for hearing aid replacement.

Thank you very much for allowing us to participate in   care. Should you have any questions, please do not hesitate to contact me.

Sincerely yours,

Douglas C. Bigelow, M.D.
Assistant Professor
Otology/Neurotology
Co-Director, Center for Cranial Base Surgery

DCB:sjc

1/29/97   _____ is in for evaluation of her right shoulder. History is that of about 5 days ago she was walking in her yard, tripped over a railroad tie and dislocated her shoulder. She was seen in the ER where she was sedated and then relocation performed. She comes in today for evaluation. Otherwise, she is healthy. No previous history of shoulder injury.

X-RAYS: X-rays confirm an anterior dislocation pre and then post reduction.

EXAM: Physical examination slightly overweight 51 year old white female. She is neurologically intact with normal deltoid function. No evidence of musculotaneous nerve injury. The shoulder is located an she has passive forward flexion of 100 degrees at which time she has pain.

IMPRESSION: Is, anterior shoulder dislocation.

PLAN: I explained to her that as we get older, the risk of re-dislocation decreases and in her situation would only be estimated at 20-30% risks of re-dislocations and need for surgery. Unfortunately, above 35, the risk of rotator cuff tearing begins to increase. At the current time we will assume that she has not torn her rotator cuff. We will put her on a standard protocol which will include gentle ROM exercises but avoiding abduction with external rotation. If she does not progress along lines that one would expect, then we will worry more about a rotator cuff tear and can always proceed to an MRI scan. LSM/afs

Typical Typed Consultation

December 9, 1996

Paul A. Lotke, M.D.
510 W. Darby Road
Havertown, Pa. 19083

Re:

Dear Paul:

As you know, I had the opportunity to see   in my
office on December 9, 1996 for another opinion regarding her left
knee.   is a very pleasant 54 year old homemaker who is active
in a variety of sports including skiing and aerobic exercise
programs. In the past she was a dancer. She's developed left knee
pain which has been present for ten years and worsened over the
summer of 1996. She possibly relates this to adding orthotics to
her shoes while walking in France. There is no specific injury and
she denies any locking although there is some intermittent
swelling. She also has a clicking sensation. Her pain is mostly
medial and worsens with squatting and twisting. She denies fevers,
chills or rash but there has been some tick exposure without joint
symptoms. Her medical history is fairly negative and she denies
allergies. She was seen by yourself and some arthritis and a
meniscal abnormality was noted and arthroscopy was suggested as an
alternative.

Physical exam of her lower extremities reveals pain free hip
motion. Her knee exam reveals a minor bilateral varus alignment.
Motion is full and there is no effusion.   On the left her
tenderness is primarily over the medial joint line which worsens
with McMurray maneuvers although I only intermittently palpate a
minor click on the medial joint line.   There is a small palpable
band along the medial retinaculum suggestive of a plica and this
too is slightly tender. There is no instability. Her right knee
is unremarkable although she does have some clicking over the
lateral meniscus with McMurray maneuvers. Neurovascular exam is
intact.

I have reviewed her MRI and there is evidence of early mild to
moderate degenerative arthritis medial greater than lateral
hemicompartment. There is also significant degenerative signal in
the medial meniscus on several cuts that appears to extend to the
inferior articular surface suggestive of degenerative tear.

In addition, there is a small posteromedial popliteal cyst.

Xrays taken today including standing films reveals a bilateral mild varus alignment. There is moderate medial joint space narrowing left greater than right although there is still approximately 20 or 30% joint space maintained. There is also some mild left sided lateral joint narrowing and lipping of her tibial spines bilaterally.

IMPRESSION: 1.   Left knee medial hemicompartment degenerative arthritis with probable superimposed degenerative tear medial meniscus and secondary Baker's cyst.
2.   Mild to moderate right knee medial hemicompartment degenerative arthritis.

Plan: I had a lengthy discussion with   and her husband and reviewed all treatment options from conservative to operative. I think arthroscopy is reasonable but I explained the limitations of arthroscopy in a knee with early arthritis. If indeed a meniscal tear is identified and resected I would expect improvement although she may need to live with some arthritic symptoms. They had some questions about skiing this season and holding off on arthroscopy and I explained the risks of this particular activity if indeed a meniscal tear is present. It is possible that she could enlarge the tear. She can continue some of her fitness routines, however, I do not anticipate any problems in that regard. They will think all the above over and contact me.

I hope you find this information useful. Thank you for your kind referral.

Sincerely yours,

Nicholas A. DiNubile, M.D.

NAD:ljk
cc: Marie Savard, M.D.

Typical Pap Test

PATIENT

AGE	SEX		COLLECTION DATE	ACCESSION DATE	REPRT DATE	ACCESSION NO.	REQUESTED BY
66	F	TEST NAME	01/11/94	01/12/94	01/18/94	0004818-0	SAVARD, MARIE

SAVARD, MARIE
191 PRESIDENTIAL BLVD. /44
BALA CYNWYD, PA 19004

		ACCOUNT NO.	FRAME	ROUTE
		22053	66806741-9	67

PATIENT'S RESULTS		
WITHIN RANGE	OUT OF RANGE	REFERENCE RANGE	UNITS

CLINICAL INFORMATION:
SOURCE...........: CERVIX, ENDOCERVIX
PATIENT HISTORY..: MENOPAUSAL

CYTOLOGY RESULTS:

PAP SMEAR MULTI SLIDE:
    INFLAMMATION:
        MILD
    VAGINAL FLORA:
        NONE SEEN
    ESTROGEN EFFECT:
        NONE
    ENDOCERVICAL SAMPLE:
        NO ENDOCERVICAL COMPONENT PRESENT.
        (ENDOCERVICAL AND/OR METAPLASTIC CELLS)

DIAGNOSIS:

BETHESDA SYSTEM:
WITHIN NORMAL LIMITS
THE ABSENCE OF ENDOCERVICAL COMPONENT IS ACCEPTABLE IN
CONDITIONS SUCH AS PREGNANCY, POST MENOPAUSE,
CERVICAL STENOSIS, OR HYSTERECTOMY.

(CLASS I — NEGATIVE FOR MALIGNANCY)

TECHNOLOGIST ID:....NCP on 13-JAN-94

*** F I N A L ***
01/18/94   Batch # 001

f o r

Thomas J. Liddy

THOMAS J. LIDDY, M.D.
LABORATORY DIRECTOR

Typical Colonoscopy

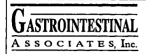

GASTROINTESTINAL
A S S O C I A T E S, Inc.

Practice Limited to Gastroenterology

Myhanh T. Bosse, M.D.
Martin Chatzinoff, M.D.
Harvey Guttmann, M.D.
Stephen E. Kaufman, M.D., F.A.C.P.
Steven C. Leskowitz, M.D.

William H. Mahood, M.D., F.A.C.P.
Anne L. Saris, M.D.
Ellen W. Shaw, M.D.
Jonathan M. Sternlieb, M.D.

July 17, 1997

Dr. Marie Savard
Presidential City
Monroe Office Center Suite 100
4000 Presidential Blvd.
Philadelphia, PA 19131-1713

RE:
DOB:
DOV: 07-07-97

Dear Marie,

had colonoscopic examination, upon your kind recommendation. The patient had the procedure performed on the 7th of July, 1997. As you know, , has generally been in relatively good health. She does have ongoing complaints of constipation and has had episodes of red rectal bleeding with a negative sigmoidoscopy, aside from the presence of hemorrhoids. She has a family history of colon cancer spanning two generations, both a paternal grandfather and her father had a colon cancer in their later years. She herself has had no abdominal pain and the bleeding that she has experienced has been bright red, primarily in the water and on the tissue paper. Her diet is a good one and she had been on FiberCon in the past but has since discontinued it. She is generally in otherwise good health, except for the presence of mitral valve prolapse.

On examination, she is a pleasant white female in no acute distress. Lungs/cardiac examination was unremarkable. Her abdomen was soft and non-tender, without hepatosplenomegaly.

After full informed consent was obtained, a colonoscopic study was performed under Demerol and Versed pre-medication, to the cecum. The mucosa was normal without colitic, diverticular or angiodysplastic change. Specifically, no neoplasia was seen. Internal hemorrhoids were present, the likely source of bleeding.

I have informed the patient of these findings, and given the fact that she has a family history of colon cancer, repeat study might be warranted in five years' time. I do not, however, believe that she fulfills the criteria of a Lynch syndrome patient, which would possibly necessitate genetic screening and/or more frequent examinations.

Thank you so much for allowing me to share in her care.

With best regards.

Harvey Guttmann, M.D.

HG/mjh
(strut707AO)

Cardiac Stress Test

PATIENT NAME: _____ AGE: ___35___ DATE: _6/3/88_____

ADDRESS: _____ IN PATIENT: _____ OUT PATIENT __X__

PH _____ ,_____ DONE BY ` Saxena _____   HEART RATE

DIAGNOSIS: dizziness DRUGS: none _____   MAXIMUM AGE PRED. _____ 188

PRE.-EXERCISE: _____ HYPERVENT. _____   85% MAXIMUM AGE PRED. 160

_____ _____   PEAK DOUBLE PRODUCT

                                             ACHIEVED MAX. HEART RATE 161

                                             THALLIUM none

PROTOCOL: BRUCE

STAGE	MPH	GRADE	MINS.	METS	HR	BP	ST SEGMENT	SYMPTOMS
BASELINE	0	0	0 mins.	1	61	100/76		
STAGE 1	1.7	10	3 mins.		120	120/76		
STAGE 2	2.5	12	3 mins.		150	130/72		dizzy
STAGE 3	3.4	14	2 mins		161	(86% predicted MHR)		dizzy
STAGE								
STAGE								
STAGE								
STAGE								

HEART RATE
PER MINUTE: |112 | 124| 120|141 |141 |150 |160 · | | | |

POST-EXERCISE DATA

TIME	BP	HR	SYMPTOMS	TIME	HR	BP	SYMPTOMS
IMMED	140/70	151					
1 Mins.		114					
2 Mins.		80					

RESULTS:

TOTAL EXERCISE TIME: _____8 minutes_____ MAX. METS 8.6 MAX. HEART RATE 161

REASON FOR TERMINATION OF TEST: fatigue with light headedness,?true vertigo(mild)

POST EXERCISE EKG: _____

INTERPRETATION:

The patient was exercised using the Bruce protocol for a toal duration of 8
minutes, and completed stage III-2.
The resting EKG revealed sinus rhythm, normal axis and intervals and nonspecific
T wave flattening in lead AVL. No significant ST segment changes were noted
throughout exercise or during the recovery phase. The tracing had returned to
baseline at 3 minutes post exercise.
Conclusion:
1. Negative treadmill exercise EKG.
2. Ph;ysiologic hemodynamic response to exercise.
3. No exercise induced chest pain or discomfort were noted. Rare ventricular
premature beat was noted in the recovery phase.

sc
6/4

                                             Saxena M.S

Heart ECHO

Name: _____ Tape: _____ 36-7 _____

Room: _____ OP _____ Age: _____

Reason for study: __Murmur__

Date: _____ 6/2/88 _____

M-Mode Results:

LV end diastolic diameter	4.7 cm.	Septal thickness	.8 cm.	Mitral valve		
LV end systolic diameter	2.9 cm.	LV posterior wall thickness	.8 cm.	Velocity (EF Slope)	nl	cm.
Fractional shortening	.38	Aortic root & valve :		Excursion	nl	cm.
		Aortic root diameter	2.4 cm.	Contour suggestive of :		
		Aortic valve separation	1.8 cm.			
Pulmonic valve		Left atrium	3.3 cm.			
Visualized: ___ no X yes				Tricuspid valve		
				Visualized: ___ no X yes		

M-Mode Conclusion:

The left ventricle is of normal size and contractility. The left
atrium is of normal size. No pericardial effusion is noted. The
aortic and mitral valves are normal.

Two Dimensional Conclusion:

The overall pattern and contraction of the left ventricle is normal. The
aortic valve is structurally normal. There is mild prolapse of the
anterior leaflet of the mitral valve seen both in the parasternal long
axis view and the four chamber view. The tricuspid valve is structurally
normal. No pericardial effusion is seen.

sc
6/4

Steven Mattan M D

232

Index

Abdominal cramps or pain, 10, 12
About.com, 61
Acid reflux, 9
Acoustic neuroma, 11
Aging, 12; skin spots (seborrheic or senile keratosis), 12
Albumin test, 84, 89
Alcohol consumption, 73, 180, 185, 190
Allergies, 10; recording, 36
AllHealth.com, 55
Alternative Health and Medicine Encyclopedia, 51
Alzheimer's Disease, 146–47
American Liver foundation, 53
Anal fissure, 11
Anemia, 11, 82, 83
Aneurysm: aortic, 10; brain, 9; sweating and, 13
Angina, 10
Anorexia nervosa, 9
Anxiety, 10, 12, 13
Aorta: aneurysm, 10; dissecting, 10
Arthritis: bone scan for, 104–5; of spine (stenosis), 12
Asthma, 9, 10

Baltimore Study on Aging, 146
Best Medical Resources on the Web, The (priory.com), 60
Bilirubin test, 85–86
Black stool, 11
Bleeding: diverticulitis, 11, 154; rectal, 11; ulcer, 11; vaginal, 11
Blood calcium level, 84–85

Blood fats test, 86–87
Blood pressure: low, 11; test, 78–79
Blood sugar: glucose test, 84; low, 12, 45–47; urinalysis, 88–89
Blood tests: chemistry, 83–86; complete blood count (CBC), 82–83; work (test), 79–82
Blood type, 38
Blood Urea Nitrogen (BUN) and Creatinine tests, 84
Bone: density test, 100–101; scan, 104–5
Brain: aneurysm, 9; tumor, 9, 12
Breast: cancer, 11, 39–40, 147, 193–94; cyst, 11; mammogram, 111–113; tissue, changes in, 11

Cancer: blood test, 85; symptoms, 9. *See also specific types*
Cardiac stress test, 96–98
Carotene, overdose, 12
CAT or CT Scan (Computed Tomography), 102–3
Chest pains, 10
Chicken pox vaccine, 69
Cholesterol: blood fat tests, 86–87; how to read tests for, 41–42
Circulatory blockage (cludication), 12
Clinton, Hilary Rodham, 25
Colon: bleeding, 11; cancer, 6–7, 90, 92, 147; colonoscopy, 92–93, 122–23; polyps, 90, 93; sigmoidoscopy, 90–91; stool or fecal samples, 89–90; spastic, 10

Colopscopy, 109

Complementary care providers, 128–29

Cough, 9, 180

Crohn's disease, 9

Denial, 13–19; embarrassment and, 17–18; inconvenient timing, 15–16; "risk blindness," 20–21; self-blame for problem, 18–19; waiting for symptoms to disappear, 16–17

Dental exam, 105–6

Depression, 8–9, 12, 13

DEXA or DXA Scan (Dual X-ray Absorptiometry Scan), 53, 100–101

Diabetes: glucose test, 84; neuropathy, 12

Diphtheria booster, 67–68

Diverticulitis, 10, 11, 154

Dizziness, 11

"Doctor within," 4

Doctors: average "panel" (caseload), xii, 4; average time spent per patient, 44–45; diagnosis, based on patient's disclosures, 117; e-mail, 134; phone calls, guidelines, 133–34; second opinion, 134–35; two-way relationship with, 136–41. *See also* *Office visits*

Dorland's Illustrated Medical Dictionary, 48

DrKoop.com, 55, 56

Drugs or medications: daily, taking, 183–84, 189; digitalis, 24; herbs and vitamins as, 129; list, recording, 36–37; minocycline, 9; overdose, 12; questions to ask when prescribed, 139–40; reactions or interactions, 12, 13; recording effectiveness or reactions, 36

Dryden, John, 179

Ear: inner, infection, 11; tumor, 11

ECG or EKG (Electrocardiogram), 95–96

Endometrial cancer biopsy, 110

Environmental or lifestyle risk factors, 73

Esophageal spasm, 10

Essential Guide to Prescription Drugs: Everything You Need to Know for Safe Drug Use (Rybacki & Long), 50–51

Evista, 148

Exercise, 182, 189

Eye: foreign body in, 9; pink (conjunctivitis), 9; redness, 9

Fasting, 12

Ferraro, Kenneth, 5

Fever, 13

Flatulence, 10

Flu shot, 68

FOBT (Fecal Occult Blood Tests), 89–90

Gallbladder: attack, 10; gallstones, 12, 148; infection, 12

Genetic risk factors, 72–73, 193–94

Gilbert's syndrome, 53–55, 85

Glaucoma, 9

Global Health Network, 61

Globulin test, 84

Harrison's Online, 62

Harrison's Principles of Internal Medicine, 48

Headaches, severe, 9

Health A to Z, 56

Health buddy, 125–26, 129, 157–58

Health calendar, 113–14, 184

Health journal, 116–21

Healthgate, 59

Index

Heart: arrhythmia, 11, 24; attack, 13; cardiac stress test, 96–98; disease in women, and HRT, 142, 144–45; ECG or EKG, 95–96; failure, 9, 11; Philbin, Regis and, 20–21, 118; transplants, 138; valve infection (subacute bacterial endocarditis), 120
Heartburn, 9, 180
Hemochromatosis, 85
Hemorrhoids, 11, 90
Hepatitis: A vaccine, 69; B vaccine, 69; symptoms, 9, 12
Herpes simplex (cold sores), 123
Hillel, xi
HIP Health Plan of New Jersey, xiii
Hippocrates, 196
Hodgkin's disease, 3
Hormone replacement therapy (HRT), 140–52
Hospital stay: chart abbreviations, 159–72; discharge planning, 174; discharge report, obtaining, 174–77; health buddy, 157–58; how to work with the staff, 172–74; note taking during, 159; problems with current care, 156–59; remaining with a loved one, 153–59
Hot flashes, 13, 142, 143
Hypercalcemia, 51–54
Hyperparathyroidism, 85
Hyperventilation, 10, 12
Hypoglycemia, 46–47, 84

Immunizations: blood tests to verify, 35; list of needed, 67–70; records, 35
Infections: bacterial, 83; blood tests for, 83; chronic, 9; septicemia, 15; staph or strep, 13–15; viral, 9, 10, 11, 83
Inflammation: blood test, 83, 84; of lining of lung or rib cage, 10

Insomnia, 13
Instincts or gut feelings, trusting, 1–8, 21–22
Intelihealth, 56–57
International Traveler's Hotline at the Centers for Disease Control, 70
Internet: e-zines, 55; Health on the Net (HON), 57; medical record services, 27–28; medical research and websites, 51–64; search engines for research versus medical sites, 53–56
iVillage, 55

Jaundice, 12, 54, 85
Johns Hopkins Family Health Book, 47
Journal of the American Medical Association, 47–48; online, 63

Kaplan-Greenfield study, 136
Koop, C. Everett, 44
Kidney disease: blood tests for, 84, 85; stones, 85; urinalysis, 88–89

Lactate Dehydrogenase (LDH) test, 85
Lactose intolerance, 10
Le Guin, Ursula, 136
Lifestyle and behavior changes, 179–81; changing habitual behaviors, 181–82; daily medication, taking, 183–84, 189; do good for others, 190; get rid of reminders of old ways, 189–90; lay in supplies for, 189; list what's holding you back, 185–88; nagging and, 184; phase-by-phase approach, 182–83; prevention, three phases of, 191–93; reward yourself, 190; scare yourself, 188–89; setting a date for, 185; support groups, 184–85; write a contract, 190

235

Liver: blood tests for, 84, 85–86; tumor, 12
Loss of appetite, 8–9
Lung: cancer, 9; collapsed, 10
Lyme vaccine, 70
Lymphoma, 9

Mammogram, 111–13
Mayo Clinic Health Letter, 57
Mayo Clinic Health Oasis, 57
Measles/mumps/rubella vaccine, 68
Medical Informal Bureau, 26
Medical Matrix, 59
Medical records: carrying personal health information list with you, 37–38, 85; consultation report, 123; copies of minor children's or aging parent's, 28–29; copying costs, 32–33; destruction of, 27; emergencies and need for, 24–25; fears of antagonizing doctor, 29–30; finding errors in, 26; follow up on requests for, 33–34; hospital discharge report, obtaining, 174–77; how to read, 40–42; immunizations, 35; importance of studying, 45–46; Internet services for, 27–28; legal entitlement to, 28, 35; locating, 30–32; lost and filling in gaps in, 35–37; ownership of, 32; sample letter requesting, 34; Savard, John, and, 24–25; SOAP notes, 124; testing results, getting copies, 38–40
"Medical Records: Getting Yours" (Samuels & Wolfe), 35
Medical testing: obtaining results, 38–40, 80–81, 91, 94–95, 96, 100, 101, 103; overcoming anxiety about, 71–72; routine exams, 74–78; routine screening tests, 78–114, *see also specific tests;*

understanding, 81, 94–95, 96, 97–98, 100, 101, 103, 104, 105, 106, 107–8, 109–10, 112–13
Mediconsult, 57
Medscape, 59–60
Melanoma, 12
Men: cholesterol readings, 86; ESR or SED rate, 83; hematocrit readings, 82; PSA Test (Prostate Specific Antigen), 107–8, 121; rectal exam, 75–76
Men's Health, 117–18
Meningitis, 9
Mental confusion, 12
Mental Health Net, 61
Merck Manual (online), 62–63
Merck Manual of Diagnosis and Therapy, 48–49
Merck Manual of Medical Information, 47
Migraine headache, 9, 12, 148
Minocycline, 9
Mitral valve prolapse, 120
Mosby's Medical Encyclopedia, 48
Mosby's Pocket Dictionary of Medicine, Nursing and Allied Health, 48
MRI Scan (Magnetic Resonance Imaging), 103–4
Multiple myeloma, 84

National Institutes of Health, 61–62
New England Journal of Medicine, 63; online, 63–64
Nightingale, Florence, 153
Numbness, 12; in feet and legs, 12
Nurses' Study, Boston, 147
Nutrition Bible, 51
Nutritional deficiencies, test for, 82

Obesity, shortness of breath and, 10
Office visits: communicating effectively, 129–30; copies of test

Index

results from, 126–28; explaining reason for visit, 122–24; health buddy, 125–26, 129; honesty during, 130–31; looking up symptoms before, 121–22; notes and tapes of, 131–32; records, bringing, 126–28; SOAP notes, 124; written list to take, 125

Oncolink, 62

OnHealth.com, 57–58

Organizations, list of, 192–93

Osler, William, 5

Osteoporosis, 84–85, 142, 145–46; test for, 100–101

Ovarian cyst, 10

Pancreas attack, 10

Pap Test, 108–10

Pelvic exam, 76–77

Personal prevention schedule: breast exam, 77–78; charting environmental risk factors, 73; charting genetic risk factors, 72–73, 193–94; general physical exam, 74–75; health calendar, 113–14, 184; immunizations, 67–70; pelvic exam, 76–77; rectal exam, 75–76; routine screening tests, 78–114, *see also specific tests*

Philbin, Regis, 20–21, 118

Phlebitis, 121–22, 148

Physical exam, general, 74–75

Physician's Desk Reference (PDR), 50

Pneumonia vaccine, 68

Polio vaccine, 69–70

Polyps, 90, 93

Postnasal drip, 9

Powell, Colin, 118

Prevention, three phases of, 191–93

Prostate: BPH (benign prostatic hypertrophy), 138; cancer, 118, 121

PSA Test (Prostate Specific Antigen), 107–8, 121

Public Citizens Publications Department, 35

Pubmed, 60.

Pulmonary embolism, 10, 13

Rectal bleeding, 11; blood tests for, 89–90

Rectal exam, 75–76

Researching conditions, diseases, injuries: books your doctor uses, 47–51; importance of knowledge, 64–66; Internet sources, 51–64; organizations, list of, 192–93

ReutersHealth.com, 54

"Risk blindness," 20–21

Ruptured organ, 10

RxList, 63

Savard, John, 24–25

Schweitzer, Albert, 1

Sedentary lifestyle, 10

SGPT and SGOT (Serum glutamine Pyruvic Transaminase and Serum Glutamine-Oxalocacetate Transaminase) test, 85

Shortness of breath, 10

Side stitch, 10

Sigmoidoscopy, 90–91

Skin: cancer, 12; change in mole or dark spot, 12

Sodium, potassium, chloride blood tests, 84

Smoking, 73, 180, 185, 189–90

Stool occult blood test, 89–90

Strawberry, Darryl, 118

Stress, 12, 13, 83

Stroke, 11, 12

Sweating, profuse, 13

Symptoms, general, to investigate, 8–13

TB, 9; skin test (PPD), 70
"Telenurse," 7
Tension headache, 9
Tetanus shots, 67–68
ThriveOnline.com, 53, 58
Thyroid blood tests, 87–88
Torsion of testicle, 7–8
Toxin exposure, 12
Travel to foreign countries, immunizations needed, 70
Treatment: aggressive versus conservative, 137–38; example, HRT, 140–52; magic bullets, lack of, 179; questions to ask regarding medication, 139–40
Triglyceride blood test, 87
Tumor: abdominal, 10; brain, 12; ear, benign, 11; fever, 7; liver, 12

Ulcer, 11
Ultrasonography (Ultrasound Scanning or Sonogram), 98
Uric Acid test, 84
Urinalysis, 88–89
Uterine cancer, 11, 141, 147–48

Uveitis, 9

Vagina, dry, 11
Vaginal bleeding (post-menopausal), 11
Vision tests, 106–7

Warning signals, 5–13
Weakness, 12
WebMD, 58
Weight: gain and bloating, 149; loss, 8–9
Women: breast exam, 77–78; cholesterol readings, 86; DEXA or DXA Scan, 100–101; endometrial biopsy, 110; ESR or SED rate, 83; health care decisions by, 117; hematocrit readings, 82; HRT, 140–52; mammogram, 111–13; menstrual history, 36; Pap Test, 108–10; pelvic exam, 76–77; rectal exam, 75–76

X-ray: Chest 9, 93–95, 97; DEXA or DXA Scan, 53, 100–101

About the Author

MARIE SAVARD, M.D. is an internationally known internist, women's health expert, and patients' rights champion. She is the creator of The Savard Health Record. Dr. Savard is also a medical writer and seminar provider who has lectured throughout the world on the principle of taking charge. She serves as medical director of the Cabrini Nursing Home.

Her past career highlights include:

•Director of the Center for Women's Health and associate professor at the Medical College of Pennsylvania/ Hahnemann University

•World Health Organization's technical advisor to the United Nations Fourth World Conference on Women (Beijing)

• *Woman's Day* magazine "Your Health" columnist

• *Philadelphia Magazine* "Top Doctor" since the 1980s

Dr. Savard received her B.S. in nursing and her M.D. degree from the University of Pennsylvania. She completed her residency in internal medicine at the Hospital of the University of Pennsylvania and completed a fellowship in general internal medicine at the University of Colorado Health Sciences Center. She serves on the trustees council of Penn Women and has served on the American Board of Internal Medicine Subcommittee on Clinical Competency in Women's Health. Dr. Savard was recently appointed by Governor Thomas Ridge to the Pennsylvania Women's Commission. To contact Dr. Savard, call toll free 1-877-SAVARDS or visit her Web site at www.drsavard.com.

SONDRA FORSYTH is a 1999 recipient of a National Magazine Award for an article on colon cancer, as well as the winner of an award from the American Digestive Health Foundation. Ms. Forsyth has served as executive editor of *Ladies' Home Journal*, and is the author or co-author of seven books. She has written extensively about health and medicine as well as other topics for the major magazines.

Ms. Forsyth holds an M.A. from Harvard University. A former ballerina, she founded the Harkness Ballet Outreach and Ballet Ambassadors in New York City and writes "The New York Dance Scene" on DanceArt.com.